BECOME YOUR CHILD'S
SLEEP COACH

Become Your Child's Sleep Coach

The Bedtime Doctor's 5-Step Guide, Ages 3–10

DR. LYNELLE SCHNEEBERG, PSYD, FELLOW, AASM

LIFE
LONG

Lifelong Books
Hachette Book Group
1290 Avenue of the Americas, New York, NY 10104

HachetteBooks.com
Twitter.com/HachetteBooks
Instagram.com/HachetteBooks

Printed in the United States of America

First Edition: September 2019

Published by Lifelong Books, an imprint of Perseus Books, LLC,
a subsidiary of Hachette Book Group, Inc. The Lifelong Books name
and logo are trademarks of the Hachette Book Group.

The Hachette Speakers Bureau provides a wide range of authors for
speaking events. To find out more, go to www.hachettespeakersbureau.com
or call (866) 376-6591.

The publisher is not responsible for websites (or their content)
that are not owned by the publisher.

Editorial production by Lori Hobkirk at the Book Factory.
Print book interior design by Cynthia Young at Sagecraft.

Library of Congress Cataloging-in-Publication Data has been applied for.

ISBNs: 978-0-7382-8556-6 (trade paperback); 978-0-7382-8555-9 (e-book)

LSC-C

10 9 8 7 6 5 4 3 2 1

To Gordon, my treasured partner in all things,
and to my beloved children, William,
Evelynne, and Marie, who inspire me every day—
may your lives be full of joy (and great sleep!)

"Yes, there is a nirvana . . .
in leading your sheep to a green pasture,
in writing the last line of your poem,
and in putting your child to sleep."

—*Kahlil Gibran*

Contents

Author's Note

The stories of children and families in this book are based on composites of people seen in the author's practice. None are based on specific people and all identifying details have been changed to protect the privacy of the children and families involved.

Foreword

Why should you become your child's sleep coach? Your child's learning and development during the preschool and elementary school years will determine how your child will do for the rest of his or her life. If your child does not achieve quality sleep during this period, this learning and development may be impaired. Memory, concentration, mood, health, and performance can all suffer. Preschool and school-age children seldom complain about sleep deprivation, but it is not hard for parents and teachers to see the results of poor sleep.

I have been treating children with sleep disorders for more than thirty years. When a family in my practice has a child with a sleep problem that would benefit from a behavioral approach, I refer that family directly to Dr. Schneeberg. She is one of only about two hundred psychologists in the country who is a Fellow of the American Academy of Sleep Medicine. Her patience and empathy, combined with her extensive clinical experience and her comprehensive training in sleep medicine, allow her to solve even the most complicated pediatric sleep problems.

She has combined this empathy, experience, and training, along with the latest sleep science, into *Become Your*

Child's Sleep Coach. This book is a tremendous resource that will teach you exactly how to solve your own child's sleep problems. Best of all, the wonderful sleep your child will achieve as a result will help your child reach his or her greatest potential.

Meir Kryger, MD

Fellow of the Royal College of Physicians of Canada
Professor, Yale School of Medicine
Author, *The Mystery of Sleep: Why a Good Night's Rest Is
    Vital to a Better, Healthier Life*

Why a Sleep Book Just for Preschool and School-Age Children?

Seven-year-old Leo had a good bedtime routine, but as soon as his parents left his bedroom, he was sure to come right out again to tell them one more thing, to get one more kiss, to give them one more hug, or to ask for one more drink of water (even though he had to pass right by a faucet with a cup to find his parents!). Leo's parents always granted these requests, hoping that once all of Leo's needs were met, he would fall asleep. However, almost every night it took more than two hours to get Leo to sleep.

Four-year-old Amanda loved her cute and colorful menagerie of stuffed animals. At bedtime, she would not get into bed unless at least a dozen of these were set up at the foot of her bed. If any of her favorites were missing, they had to be found. If any of them fell over, they had to be set up again before she would lie down. Once her stuffed animals were settled, Amanda's mother would leave Amanda's room to put the baby to sleep, and Amanda's father would rub her back and read to her until she fell asleep.

Her father stopped reading when he thought Amanda was asleep, but Amanda often sat right up again to ask him to keep reading. Reading her to sleep often took well over an hour. During the middle of the night, each time Amanda awoke, she would call her father back to reset her stuffed animals or to read again. This happened many times each night, and both Amanda and her father were becoming very sleep-deprived.

Do these stories sound familiar? If bedtime is a struggle in your home, this book will teach you how to improve your child's sleep with a proven five-step plan.

Parents of babies and toddlers have a myriad of books to help them improve their child's sleep, but most books have one chapter or less on older children. You, the parent of a preschool or elementary school-aged child, may be suffering in silence. You may even be embarrassed to admit that your children still have sleep issues. If so, you will be relieved to discover you have plenty of company.

How much company? Let's explore some data from the National Sleep Foundation (NSF). The NSF commissions a "Sleep in America" poll on different sleep-related topics each year. The most recent national poll studying sleep in children aged ten and younger was completed in 2004.*

---

*"2004 Sleep in America Poll," from National Sleep Foundation (Washington, DC: 2004).

A random national sample of 1,473 parents of children ages ten and younger were asked about their children's sleep behaviors, routines, and environments.

This poll revealed some eye-opening statistics:

- Almost three out of four parents reported that their child's sleep needed improvement.

- Sixty-nine percent reported that their child had sleep problems a few nights each week.

- More than half of the preschooler parents reported that their children stalled about going to bed, and one-quarter of them noted that their children seemed overtired during the day. Almost 20 percent reported that their children had difficulty waking in the morning.

- Forty-two percent of parents with school-aged children reported their children stalled about going to bed, and almost 20 percent had difficulty waking in the morning.

- Forty-three percent of parents of toddlers and pre-schoolers are present when their children fall asleep, and 23 percent of parents of school-aged children are present when their children fall asleep.

Convinced now that you are not alone? Ready to do something about it? You may be ready to help your child become a better sleeper, but you may feel unsure about how to proceed without causing lots of stalling, anxiety, and tears. You may even worry that you might cause some type of trauma for your child, so you have considered seeking help from a professional sleep coach.

However, you may have several concerns about this type of help. First, you may worry that sleep training is too expensive. Sleep coaches can charge up to several hundred dollars per hour to work with families, and several hours are often required. Other sleep coaches recommend in-home overnight visits that may be quite expensive, too, and several nights may be needed. Next, you may think that you have already tried everything a sleep coach would suggest. And finally, you may worry that sleep training will involve a cry-it-out approach that you are unwilling to try.

However, parents actually make wonderful sleep coaches for their children once they understand the simple reasons sleep difficulties start in the first place and recognize they can learn exactly how to manage these problems. Countless numbers of parents, with all of the right intentions, make some very common mistakes at bedtime, ones that are almost guaranteed to make their children poor sleepers. Parents make these mistakes out of frustration and, frankly, even out of desperation, but these result in children who stay awake longer at bedtime and, perhaps even worse, stay awake for long periods during the night.

Once you learn how to use this book's five-step plan to help your child fall asleep quickly, easily, and independently, you will become a confident sleep coach. This book takes all the guesswork out of this quest, and you can feel confident about trying this approach because it is based on solid behavioral research and extensive clinical experience.

Let's start with a questionnaire (page 6) to help you decide whether your child would benefit from sleep coaching. Place a check mark next to any of the following questions that are true for your child.

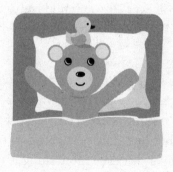

PARENT QUESTIONNAIRE

Please check the questions below that are true for your child:

___ Does your child stall or get more energetic at bedtime?

___ Does your child become clingy or anxious at bedtime?

___ Does your child complain of feeling sick at bedtime (when he or she seemed fine earlier)?

___ Does your child refuse to sleep in his or her own room at bedtime?

___ Do you ever let your child stay up very late or fall asleep in your bed to avoid bedtime battles?

___ Does your child find many reasons to call you back into the bedroom after the bedtime routine is over (for a cup of water, another hug, an escorted trip to the bathroom, or just "one more thing")?

___ Does your child come out of his or her room to find you after the bedtime routine is over?

___ Do you frequently stay with your child to get him or her to sleep?

___ Does your child fall asleep easily at bedtime when you are nearby but wake often during the night?

___ Does your child fall asleep only if electronics are on (TV, smartphone, tablet)?

___ Do you ever find yourself getting upset at bedtime despite your best intentions?

___ Are you afraid to set limits at bedtime because your child might disturb others?

___ Does your child get less sleep than you'd like because the bedtime routine takes so long?

___ Does your child fall asleep more easily for one parent? For a grandparent? For a sitter?

___ Do you avoid dates with your spouse because your child will not fall asleep when you are away?

___ Does your child slip into your bed (or a sibling's bed) during the night?

If you put a check next to some (or most!) of these questions, you are definitely not alone. Read on for the help you need!

The five-step plan in this book will soon put your family on the path to great sleep. This plan will help you teach your child to be a great sleeper so that he or she can fall asleep easily and independently in his or her own bedroom and stay there throughout the night.

Sleep problems in children are very common and often have a major impact on the family, but they are also highly and (good news!) fairly easily treatable. Believe it or not, about *80 percent of parents with preschoolers* say that their child's sleep needs improvement. Almost all children resist going to bed, but the way you manage this and other bedtime issues makes all the difference.

Your family probably does not need this book if your bedtime routine is working well for your child as well as for you and your spouse or partner. More specifically, if your child is falling asleep quickly, has only infrequent nocturnal awakenings, and is waking up rested each day, just keep on doing what you are doing!

Also, this book may not be helpful for families who prefer to co-sleep (sleep together in the same bed) each night. However, this book will help your family if you are co-sleeping *only because you desperately want your child to go to sleep* and you haven't been able to figure out how to break the habit. This is called "reactive co-sleeping" (as opposed to "intentional co-sleeping"), and *Become Your Child's Sleep Coach* has a plan that will help you to gently teach your child how to fall asleep independently in his or her own bed every night.

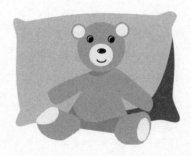

PART I

The Benefits of Sleep Coaching

"People who say they sleep like a baby
usually don't have one."

—*Leo J. Burke*

Before you use the five-step guide to help your child become a great sleeper, let's briefly review the basics and benefits of sleep coaching. In Chapter 1, you will review how much sleep your child really needs. In Chapter 2, you will learn how sleep problems get started in the first place, and in Chapter 3 you will explore the many benefits of sleep coaching for your child and for your entire family.

1

How Much Sleep Does My Child Really Need?

Five-year-old Mira was not getting nearly enough sleep each night. Her mother was an emergency room physician who worked a night shift and left for work around 10:15 p.m. each night. Even though Mira had a great bedtime routine that wrapped up around 8 p.m., Mira would call her mother back for all kinds of reasons so that she would have more time with her mother before she left for work. Mira was losing about two hours of sleep each night.

How much sleep does your child really need? The amount of sleep needed for a child does vary, but in general, pre-schoolers need ten to thirteen hours of sleep (including naps), and school-aged children need nine to eleven hours.*

---

*M. Hirshkowitz, K. Whiton, & S. M. Albert, et al., "National Sleep Foundation's Sleep Time Duration Recommendations: Methodology and Results Summary," *Sleep Health*, 1, no. 1 (2015): 40–43.

What is a simple way to know if your child is getting enough sleep? You should not have to wake your three- to ten-year-old child in the morning. He or she should wake spontaneously.

If you would like to review more specific information on how much sleep is recommended for preschoolers and school-aged children, please visit the National Sleep Foundation's website for a very useful chart.

2

How Sleep Problems
Start in the First Place

Remember the story of Amanda in the prologue who needed a dozen stuffed animals and the sound of her father's voice reading to her for more than an hour to fall asleep each night? Before we review the five steps in the plan, let's first explore how bedtime problems begin in the first place. Before Amanda's father became a parent, he may have imagined a simple, cozy bedtime routine. Perhaps he envisioned serving milk and warm peanut butter cookies in the kitchen, helping his daughter put on cozy flannel pajamas, and then spending a few minutes curled up together reading her favorite story. Her eyelids would soon begin to droop, and he would tuck her in, tiptoe out of her room, and join his wife in the living room for a glass of wine and a movie.

The reality in Amanda's home, and yours, may look far different, however. Your current routine may last hours, beginning with stalling and protesting as soon as it is time to go upstairs after the bedtime snack. Once your child has finished a bath, it might be quite the struggle to get him or her to put on pajamas. And once your child is in bed, he or she might insist on a long back rub until he or she is deeply asleep. If you do manage to slip out once your child seems to have drifted off, you may find that he or she soon wakes up and begins calling you back for what often seems like an almost infinite variety of requests: another drink of water, a bigger stuffed animal, or a closet "monster check."

Once you finally do get your child to sleep and you settle into your favorite spot on the living room sofa, you have learned from past experience that your child is likely to come and find you to ask for "one more thing." He or she is sure to tell you that he or she really, really, *really* misses you and needs one more hug and kiss. You always quickly comply, thinking that if you grant all your child's requests, he or she will *finally* be able to fall asleep. But as you probably suspect, and may have experienced, this is usually not the case.

You might also have found that if you do try to set limits at bedtime, your child becomes angry or distressed, and since you do not want him or her to be upset just before falling asleep, you give up and give in, night after night.

Bedtime problems and limit-setting issues are even more common if a child has any type of special need or medical issue, or if parents feel a bit guilty about the quantity or quality of time they are able to spend with their children. Finally, many parents are not sure how to set consistent limits at bedtime if their child is hyperactive or anxious.

Why Does My Child Have Sleep Problems?

Before you begin coaching your child to be a great sleeper, let's examine the two most common mistakes you might be making at bedtime:

- staying with your child until he or she falls completely and deeply asleep

- not setting clear limits at bedtime by allowing too many extra requests or trips out of the room after the bedtime routine is over

You might be making these mistakes with all of the right intentions, of course, but they can result in a child who is a very poor sleeper. Let's explore why.

Mistake #1: Staying with Your Child Until He or She Falls Completely Asleep

All parents know and love the joys of bedtime snuggling. However, the first mistake you might be making is staying with your child every night (or almost every night) until he or she falls completely asleep instead of gradually teaching your child how to self-comfort and fall asleep independently.

Staying with your child at bedtime teaches your child to depend on your presence in order to fall asleep. Sometimes you might provide even more than just your presence. You might be offering many additional comforting behaviors such as holding your child's hand, singing a certain song over and over, or rubbing your child's back for long periods. Since these behaviors help your child fall asleep and eventually become necessary each and every night, they are sometimes called "sleep crutches" or "sleep props" (or even the unwieldy "negative sleep-onset associations").

No matter what these are called, they all refer to the fact that your child has not learned to fall asleep independently. For example, your child may have learned to fall asleep easily while you read a book aloud. Or perhaps your child can fall asleep quickly if allowed to twirl a strand of your hair or hold your hand. Your child may have learned to fall asleep only on the living room couch while you and your spouse watch a show, or your preschool child may have learned to fall asleep only while drinking milk from a cup or bottle you frequently refill for her.

Children who have become used to this type of comforting often have a difficult time falling asleep at bedtime. This is because sometimes you might try to leave before your child is fully asleep, and your child must stay "on guard" to make sure you remain nearby. Because you might try to leave before your child is deeply asleep, he or she might also ask to do things that involve a physical connection with you so that it is much more difficult for you to slip away too soon (like asking to hold your hand).

This type of comforting at bedtime is also problematic because most children wake up several times during the night, usually at the end of a sleep cycle. Since your child has become used to falling asleep only with your help, your child will have a problem getting back to sleep whenever he or she awakens, whether this happens the first time you try to slip out, or later during the night.

When your child awakens and you are no longer available, your child doesn't have what he or she needs to fall back to sleep. If you are no longer nearby to provide the back rub or the hand-holding he or she requires, your child will call out or come to find you. He or she must try to recreate the same conditions that were present at bedtime.

Your child cannot fall asleep independently without these things, and only you can provide them. This problem results in extended bedtime routines as well as frequent and long night awakenings. This situation also leads to exhausted parents and frustrated children.

Adults have preferred ways of falling asleep, too, of course. You probably like a certain type of pillow or want to sleep on a certain side of the bed. If you woke up at night and your pillow was gone or you found yourself in a different place, you might also have difficulty returning to sleep. If your child awakens and you are gone, he or she will have the same kind of difficulty returning to sleep, too. If your child fears that you will leave before he or she is asleep, your child will try to remain alert and watchful just as you would if you feared that someone might take your pillow as you were trying to fall asleep.

However, this type of parental comforting can be gradually replaced with behaviors that allow your child to self-soothe and with security objects that can always be present for your child. If you woke up and found that your pillow was gone but you could easily reach over and find it again, you would retrieve it quickly and fall right back to sleep. If your child wakes up and finds that he or she has everything necessary to self-comfort, your child will soon be able to fall back to sleep quickly and independently, too, after some coaching and practice.

It's also important to put a child to bed each night in his or her own room. Your child might be able to fall asleep quickly in your bed, even without you in it, because he or she knows you will be coming to bed later. Your child also might be able to fall asleep easily on the living room sofa while you do chores in the kitchen or watch TV nearby, but when he or she wakes up in his or her own bed later after being carried there, your child will almost always call out or come to find you. Sometimes your child might even go back to the living room sofa during the night after an awakening and turn on the TV again to try to get back to sleep. Your child has had no practice falling asleep in his or her own cozy and quiet room. It would be disconcerting for you to wake up somewhere other than where you fell asleep, so be sure to teach your child to fall asleep only in his or her own room.

Mistake #2: Not Setting Clear Limits by Allowing Too Many Extra Requests

If your child doesn't know how to fall asleep independently, he or she will try to put off falling asleep as long as possible. So, the second mistake you might be making is allowing too many extra requests or trips out of the room after the bedtime routine ends. In this book, these extra requests are referred to as "callbacks," and these trips out of the room are referred to as "curtain calls."

Callbacks refer to all of those additional requests or demands your child makes when the bedtime routine is supposed to be over. Your child might want to tell you one more story about the day or ask for one more glass of water. Your child might want multiple escorted trips to the bathroom or ask to give you another hug and kiss. Your child might tell you something hurts, even when nothing seemed to be bothering him or her just before bedtime. Your child might begin to make lots of noise or jump up and down on the bed so you will come quickly back to his or her room. Your child might even exhibit fearful behaviors such as clinging, crying, or talking about seeing monsters (or other frightening things).

Curtain calls are those trips out of the room your child makes to find you in order to make these same types of requests. Your child might want to give you one more hug, let you know that he or she already misses you, or tell you a funny story about something that happened at school that day.

You might be allowing these callbacks and curtain calls in the mistaken belief that once your child has everything he or she needs, your child will finally fall asleep. In reality, your child learns there is no clear endpoint to the bedtime routine. When you keep responding to all these requests, you are actually (but unintentionally, of course) rewarding your child for staying awake!

Your child loves being with you and naturally wants as much time with you as possible (even when it's long past time to go to sleep). When you combine this with the fact that your child does not yet know how to fall asleep independently, your child will try to extend the bedtime routine as long as possible (far past the point of exhaustion) in order to put off the task of learning to fall asleep independently.

Note that these kinds of behaviors usually *do not* indicate that your child has some kind of anxiety-related issue. Instead, your child is just demonstrating that he or she does not yet know how to fall asleep independently. Your child will try all of these behaviors to keep you nearby because that's the only way he or she knows how to get the job done. Typical callbacks and curtain calls might include the following:

- asking for one more story, one more hug, or one more blanket tuck
- bypassing a water cup in the bathroom to ask you for water
- asking for something else to eat, even after having a substantial bedtime snack
- asking for one more escorted trip to the bathroom
- reporting a bad dream after only a brief period of sleep
- reporting a monster sighting or a strange noise
- telling you that he or she feels sick or that something hurts (when nothing seemed to be the matter just before bedtime)
- making so much noise with a sibling that you have to come back to their room
- insisting on falling asleep next to you on the sofa or in your bed

Until you teach your child to fall asleep independently, and until you set consistent limits at bedtime, your child will have difficulty falling and staying asleep.

Sleep coaches often work with families on these issues, but sleep coaches can be expensive. Instead of spending hundreds or even thousands of dollars for sleep training, you can learn how to teach your child to become a great sleeper by addressing these two mistakes with the easy five-step plan in Part II of this book.

3

How Sleep Training Benefits
Your Child and the Whole Family

Helping your child become a great sleeper will result in benefits to both your child and to your whole family.

How Sleep Training Benefits Your Child

Let's first talk about the many benefits for your child. These benefits are wide-ranging and significant.

Your Child Will Obtain
More and Better-Quality Sleep

Many families, without intending to, have bedtime routines that take hours. This happens for the two reasons we've covered: children who do not know how to fall asleep independently will try *anything* to put this task off, and bedtime routines without a clear endpoint result in many extra requests from children. When you take the time to teach your child to self-comfort, and when you use a bed-time routine with a very clear endpoint, your child will learn to accept the end of the routine and get down to the business of actually falling asleep much more quickly, thus obtaining much more of the quality sleep he or she needs.

Your Child Will Feel Safer and More Relaxed at Bedtime

In some families, the bedtime routine goes on for an extended period and the endpoint often becomes, unfortunately, the moment when the parent becomes frustrated and angry. This will not be the case for your family because, by using the five-step plan in this book, your child will learn exactly what marks the end of the bedtime routine and will know how to relax into sleep independently. You will also learn how to give your child's bedtime routine a clear endpoint and will manage callbacks and curtain calls with a simple technique, the "Bedtime Ticket." We will review Bedtime Tickets and how to use them in later chapters.

Your child benefits from knowing that you are in charge. Your child may even feel less safe without good boundaries at bedtime, so creating structure and setting consistent limits is actually very reassuring for your child. Think about which kind of classroom you would want your child in. One in which children had most of the control? Or one in which a loving, firm teacher had the control? Your child will feel much less anxious and will fall asleep more easily when he or she knows that you are in control at bedtime.

Your child may also find it confusing and upsetting if he or she cannot predict what the rules will be. In some families, children may find the bedtime rules change from night to night or notice that their parents seem to have more patience on one night than on another. This can be disconcerting for children because, on some nights, their parents are overly accommodating and, on other nights, their parents might quickly become angry at bedtime. When parents are clear and consistent about the rules and the bedtime routine, a child can give up on trying to figure out what the "rules of the night" are and will learn how to relax more quickly into sleep.

Your Child Will Fall Asleep for Other Caregivers

Once your child can fall asleep independently, your child will be able to go to sleep more easily for a babysitter, a relative, or a friend. Your child will also be able to comfortably go on sleepovers or sleep-away summer camp, or spend the night at a friend's or relative's home.

Your Child Will Learn to Stay in Bed All Night

Children who fall asleep in their own beds quickly and independently night after night are far more likely to fall quickly back to sleep in their own beds after any awakenings at night because they will have had a lot of practice doing this successfully at bedtime. Many people, even adults, actually sleep best when sleeping alone. Overnight sleep studies show that people who sleep alone have fewer awakenings and change positions less often than those who sleep with someone. Sleeping independently is not something to be avoided; it often results in better sleep.

Your Child Will Learn to Accept Limit-Setting

There are two things children benefit from learning as they grow up: that they will not always get their way and that they sometimes have to do things they do not want to do. Setting limits at night helps your child learn both of these important concepts.

If your child has trouble with limit-setting at bedtime and is making lots of callbacks and curtain calls, his or her bedtime difficulties will improve when you learn how to set clear limits at bedtime in Chapter 7. You may be a parent who has no difficulty setting limits during the day, but you may have much more trouble doing so at bedtime because all parents hope that bedtime will be a time completely free of any tears or power struggles.

During the day, you probably would not ever allow your child to play with matches or to run in a parking lot. You would never consider letting your child have lots of sugary snacks before dinner or decide whether or not to have a bath. You would not allow your child to yell and scream in a restaurant or decide whether to go to school or not. If your child complained or cried about these rules, you would most likely ignore these protests. If you are firm about these kinds of daytime rules, then you can set firm rules at nighttime, too, and you can try not to worry about a few tears here and there. Try to leave behind any guilt about a gentle, age-appropriate bedtime routine with limits.

Your Child Will Learn to Follow Simple Rules

Kids are born rule-testers, but a very critical developmental task for your child is to learn how to follow simple rules. Setting limits at bedtime helps your child learn to respond to limits in other areas, too. For example, if you wouldn't allow your child to get seven kinds of candy when you go grocery shopping, then you might agree that it isn't good for your child to make seven callbacks or curtain calls when the bedtime routine ends.

If you find yourself complaining to your pediatrician or to other parents that your child *demands* a certain food, *insists* on a certain type of cup, or *accepts* only one parent at bedtime, you may not yet have established the kind of bedtime rules that will lead to your child becoming a great sleeper. You may have become caught in the trap of doing what your child wants, not what your child needs, if you want him or her to become a good sleeper.

Your Child Will Have Fewer Behavioral Problems

Good sleep is essential for good health. Having a long, drawn-out bedtime routine results in sleep loss. Sleep-deprived kids can be irritable kids with short fuses who may have behavioral problems during the day. Typical behavioral problems might include aggressiveness, defiance, impulsivity, hyperactivity, and frequent tantrums.[*]

Your Child Is Less Likely to Develop Anxiety or Depression

Kids who obtain adequate, consolidated sleep are less likely to develop depression and anxiety later in life. A lack of sleep can lead to more negative emotions and can also make it harder for your child to take pleasure in positive experiences and to remember these good experiences later.[†]

---

[*]Elsie M. Taveras, et al., "Prospective Study of Insufficient Sleep and Neurobehavioral Functioning Among School-Age Children," *Academic Pediatrics*, 17, no. 6 (2017): 625–632.

[†]Cara Palmer and Candice Alfano, "Sleep and Emotion Regulation: An Organizing, Integrative Review," *Sleep Medicine Reviews*, 31, no. 2 (2016): 6–16.

Your Child Will Have Fewer
Sleep Deprivation–Related Problems

Nightmares, night terrors, sleepwalking, and bedwetting are much more common if a child is sleep deprived, so getting the right amount of sleep is important for these reasons, too. Chapter 11 has more information on these issues.

Your Child's Attention
Will Improve During the Day

A child with insufficient sleep may develop learning difficulties because it can be much harder to focus and pay attention during the day's activities with too little sleep. Some children with poor sleep may even be diagnosed with attention deficit and hyperactivity disorder (ADHD) and may be put on medication when they might simply need more and better-quality sleep. (Sleep apnea should also be ruled out when a diagnosis of ADHD is being considered, too. See Chapter 9 for more information on this.)

Adequate sleep helps your child organize, remember, and recall what he or she has learned during the day. Kids who sleep better usually have better grades. Finally, remember that your child's teacher will have a much easier and more enjoyable time working with your well-rested child!*

---

*Fallone Gahan, Christine Acebo, et al., "Experimental Restriction of Sleep Opportunity in Children: Effects on Teacher Ratings," *Sleep*, 28, no. 12 (2005): 1561–1567.

Your Child's Health and Development Will Improve

A sleep-deprived child may have lowered immune function.* Children who do not obtain enough sleep at night for long periods may also have a higher risk of becoming overweight or obese.†

Your Child Will Learn to Fall Asleep Without Medications

Many parents whose children have sleep problems ask their pediatrician about whether they should try a mild sleep medication to improve their sleep. A study in 2007 reported that more than 80 percent of pediatric patients with insomnia were prescribed a sleep medication.‡ Probably the most common medications tried are melatonin, diphenhydramine (Benadryl), and clonidine. However, these

---

*C. E. Gamaldo, A. K. Shaikh, and J. C. McArthur, "The Sleep-Immunity Relationship," *Neurologic Clinics*, 30, no. 4 (2012): 1313–1343.

†Alison L. Miller, Julie C. Lumeng, et al., "Sleep Patterns and Obesity in Childhood," *Current Opinion in Endocrinology and Diabetes and Obesity*, 22, no. 1 (2015): 41–47.

‡Sasko D. Stojanovski, S. Rafia, et al., "Trends in Medication Prescribing for Pediatric Sleep Difficulties in US Outpatient Settings," *Sleep*, 30, no. 8 (2007): 1013–1017.

medications might not work well, might not keep a child asleep all night, or might stop working altogether after a short period of time. They may also have unpleasant or undesirable side effects (such as disturbing dreams) or may have carryover effects on your child the next day (such as grogginess or fatigue). Many sleep problems in children are due to behavioral sleep issues that can be solved without using medication at all, but by using only behavioral strategies, such as the the five-step plan in this book.

Your Child Will Self-Comfort at Night After an Awakening

Children who don't know how to fall asleep independently at bedtime often express many nighttime fears and often become anxious fairly quickly after an awakening. Your child will soon learn how to put himself or herself back to sleep during the night and this will lead to far fewer nighttime fears.

Your Child Will Manage Daytime Stress Better

Children who learn how to self-comfort at bedtime can use these skills to feel calm and relaxed in other situations during the day, too. These kids often have better coping and social skills than peers who can't settle themselves at bedtime.

Your Child Will Learn to
Fall Asleep Independently

Some parents think their child will eventually outgrow the desire to sleep near a parent (and some children do), but there are a significant number of older children who have become so used to sleeping near a parent that they still cannot sleep well any other way.

Think about it: Would you ever "outgrow" your need to sleep with a pillow? Probably not, of course. Nevertheless, you may have actually become one of your child's "pillows," in a way. Not every child chooses a certain age or time to begin sleeping independently and some children may need a bit of help to do this. Some children who are unable to sleep independently can develop significant difficulties with insomnia and can even develop social or academic difficulties due to their inability to sleep on their own.

Studies have indicated a significant rise in co-sleeping among older children. According to Parenting's Mom-Connection, a surprising 45 percent of moms let their eight- to twelve-year-olds sleep with them from time to time, and 13 percent permit it every night.* Many of these parents are co-sleeping with their children only because they do not know how to help them to sleep well any other way.

---

*Nancy Gottesman, "Co-Sleeping with a Tween," Parenting, https://www.parenting.com/article/co-sleeping-with-a-tween.

Your Child Will Learn to Consider Everyone's Needs

Teaching your child that you and your spouse set the rules at bedtime demonstrates to your child that he or she is only one member of your family and that every member of the family has valid needs. Your child will learn that he does not run the household (and, therefore, does not run the classroom, grocery store, movie theater, or restaurant). This concept helps your child learn that the larger world has boundaries, rules, and routines that often must be followed. If your child does not learn these concepts, your child may have some social difficulties down the road, and others may find your child difficult to be around.

Your Child Will Have Good Sleep Skills for Life

Creating good bedtime routines when your child is young helps your child develop and maintain good sleep as he or she grows into a teen and an adult. Children who are poor sleepers often grow up to be adults with insomnia. Once your child knows how to fall asleep independently, he or she will be a confident sleeper for the rest of his or her life. Learning how to self-comfort and relax into sleep independently is an incredibly valuable skill, and as a parent who becomes your child's sleep coach, you will feel so gratified once you have taught your child how to do this!

How Sleep Training Benefits
the Whole Family

Helping your child become a great sleeper will bring so many benefits to you, your spouse, and your entire family. The following are just some of these benefits.

You Will Be Able to Give Each Child
Some Attention at Bedtime

You will eventually *have to* establish a good bedtime routine and set limits, if you have more than one child. For example, it's fairly easy to lie down with one child until he or she falls asleep, but what happens when you have another child? And what happens to the "family bed" when there are eventually four or five members of the family?

You and Your Spouse Will Have
More Quality Time Together

If your child learns to fall asleep quickly and independently, your relationship with your spouse is likely to improve. You and your spouse will have more time to enjoy each other, to spend time on your favorite activities, to read or study, to catch up on projects, to go out with your friends, or to simply relax and recharge. Needing an hour or two at the end of the day isn't selfish; it's essential for you two as a couple.

Your child will see that your marriage is important to the two of you. (And you won't end up falling asleep unintentionally in your child's room each night at your child's bedtime!)

You and Your Spouse Will Have Your Bedroom Back

If you teach your child how to sleep independently in her own bed, you are also sending a strong, positive message about how the family structure works. In other words, allowing your child to literally separate you and your spouse by sleeping between the two of you or to replace your spouse in the bed (since one spouse often eventually leaves the bedroom to seek better sleep elsewhere) does send a powerful message. If this is not the message you want to teach your child, consider helping her learn how to fall asleep independently by using the five-step plan in this book.

Your Home Will Feel More Peaceful in the Evening

You may find that your new bedtime routine results in a home with far fewer bedtime battles, so your home is likely to feel much more peaceful and relaxed. (And who wouldn't sign up for that?)

You and Your Spouse Will Be Better Rested

You are a better parent when you are rested, and it is more difficult to be well rested when your child is not sleeping well. Just as your child does not function at her best when she is sleep deprived, neither will you. You and your family members are all likely to be happier when you are all sleeping better.

PART II

The Five-Step Guide

*"There is a time for many words,
and there is also a time for sleep."*
—*Homer*

This book has a five-step guide to help you coach your child to be a great sleeper. We will work together to complete these five steps, and each step will lead you and your child closer to the final goal: great sleep for your child and for the whole family! Here are the steps:

1. Prepare your child's bedroom for great sleep
2. Use the 5B Bedtime Routine every night
3. Teach your child to self-comfort as you work your way out of the room
4. Limit callbacks and curtain calls
5. Manage night and early morning wakings

Let's get started!

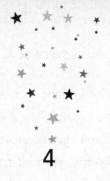

4

STEP 1:
Prepare Your Child's Bedroom
for Great Sleep

Four-year-old Tasha's mom often worried about how little sleep Tasha was getting. She worked hard to make Tasha's bedroom a perfect sleep environment. She added a sound machine that played ocean waves and an essential oil diffuser that wafted the scent of lavender flowers near Tasha's bed. She replaced the white lightbulbs in Tasha's room with pink ones that cast a warm glow. She added a star projector that made the constellations revolve on Tasha's bedroom ceiling and gave her a weighted blanket along with lots of special pillows.

While there is no problem with doing one or two things to improve your child's bedroom, sometimes parents make far too many changes. Your child can become accustomed to having all of these "sleep aids" available every night, and this can make it hard for your child to sleep anywhere else without them. Your child might even ask to take them along if he or she sleeps at a cousin's home or has a sleepover at a best friend's house. Even the nicest hotels won't have these items, so you may also find yourself trying to pack them up for a family trip.

Once you consider the pros and cons, you are likely to agree that it is best to help your child learn to fall asleep easily and quickly in a simple, basic bedroom. In this chapter, you will review the changes you can make to your child's room to ensure that you will be a successful sleep coach. You will read about exactly what to add and what to remove, and can use the comprehensive checklist at the end of this chapter to make sure you have not missed anything.

Items to Remove

Electronics

Seven-year-old Armand loved to play with a smartphone in bed at night until he fell asleep. He became so used to this (and became so angry when his mother tried to take it away) that his mother eventually had to make sure the phone ran out of power each night around bedtime so that Armand would go to sleep. However, Armand eventually learned to act like he was asleep until everyone else in his family was sleeping, and then he would search out another smartphone to use during the night. Armand became very sleep deprived, and his mother had a very difficult time waking him up for school each morning.

The first order of business is to get rid of any electronics in your child's room (TV, smartphones, tablets, laptop computers, or video game systems) and move them to another room such as a spare room, a playroom, or the living room. If you want your child to become a great sleeper and want to avoid bedtime battles, these really have no place in your child's bedroom.

If your child already needs these to fall asleep, you have probably already noticed he or she often wants these to be on all night. If you turn them off when you go to bed, you may find that your child gets up to turn them on again (or calls out to ask you to) if he or she awakens at night. All children awaken several times a night, usually at the end of a sleep cycle, so you want to avoid having these electronics on at bedtime.

Studies show that children who have a TV in their bedroom are more likely to get less sleep, go to sleep later, and have more nighttime fears.* These devices can also become problematic "sleep crutches" at bedtime for children, and as

---

* "2004 Sleep in America Poll," National Sleep Foundation (Washington, DC: 2004).

noted before, children may need them to be on all night in order to stay asleep.

If you are unwilling to remove electronics from your child's bedroom entirely, at least turn them off one hour before the bedtime routine begins and keep them off all night. Also, make them inoperable at bedtime by removing remote controllers, game consoles, DVDs and so on, keeping these under your control. (You might have to become very skilled at locking these up or putting them somewhere that your child cannot find them; kids are experts at knowing where you stash things!)

In addition, as your children get older, you will have a harder and harder time controlling the use of these devices, especially if they are in their bedroom. Please consider getting rid of them now so your child will be a great sleeper for years to come.

It is often very useful to have some house rules for the use of electronics in your home. Here is a suggested contract you may wish to customize and adopt for your family.

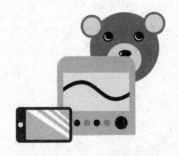

HOUSE RULES
FOR ELECTRONIC DEVICES

We know if we use electronics less in the evening, we will have more time for being together as a family. We will have more time for reading, playing board and card games, enjoying a variety of hobbies and creative activities, and, very importantly, sleeping!

We also know that electronics can interfere with sleep because the light from screens can make our brains think it is still daytime. We don't use electronic devices in bed because calls, messages, notifications, games, and videos are hard to ignore when everything is dark and quiet.

With this in mind, we agree to the following house rules for evening and nighttime use of electronics:

- We agree to use the "night mode" on our electronics from dinnertime until breakfast time.

- We agree to turn devices off one hour before bedtime and to leave them off until after breakfast.

- We agree to leave our devices overnight in our parent's bedroom or in the main living area of our home (kitchen or living room).

Smartphones

Smartphones deserve special mention because children can become so attached to them. Ideally, you would teach your child that smartphones are to be turned off at least one hour before bedtime and left overnight in the kitchen, living room, or master bedroom.

There are several issues with smartphone use at bedtime. Smartphone use is likely to lead to less sleep, poorer sleep quality, and daytime sleepiness.* A smartphone screen is confusing for your child's brain at bedtime as well because it mimics daylight and may fool your child's brain into thinking it is not time for sleep. A smartphone also provides your child with unlimited entertainment and allows your child to interact for long periods with friends, too, when it is time to be relaxing into sleep. You can always provide your child with a regular alarm clock if he or she uses a smartphone as an alarm clock.

Anything That Turns Off After a Set Period of Time

Remove anything that turns off after a set period of time (e.g., music players or star projectors that shut off after twenty

---

*B. Carter, P. Rees, et al., "Association between portable screen-based media device access or use and sleep outcomes: A systematic review and meta-analysis," *JAMA Pediatrics*, 170, no. 12 (2016): 1202–1208.

minutes). These can trigger an awakening for a child when they shut off. Also, if these do turn off later, the bedroom will not look and sound the same in the middle of the night as it did at bedtime. This can be disorienting for a child. For example, a child might want his star projector turned back on when he awakens and this can lead to a longer awakening. Remember, you should not turn off anything in your child's room when you go to bed for the same reasons.

Five-year-old Liam had a nightlight that turned off after forty-five minutes. His parents had to stay close by when he was falling asleep because if the nightlight clicked off just before he fell asleep, he would wake up again. If it turned off just after he fell asleep, he was also likely to wake up right away and call his parents back to his room to turn it back on. His parents learned that they should replace this nightlight with one that cast a soft glow all night.

Pets

You may want to discourage a pet from sleeping in your child's room. A pet may cause your child to awaken for many reasons: by making a noise, by leaving the bedroom, by waking the child to be fed, or by needing to be let out. Your child may also become dependent on having the pet nearby to fall asleep and pets may not always be willing to stay in your child's room at bedtime or throughout the night.

Three-year-old Iona loved her cat, Tigger, so much that she developed a way to keep Tigger in her room all night. She kept a container of cat treats on her bedside and gave Tigger a treat frequently during the evening. But once Iona fell asleep, Tigger would continue to request a treat many times each night by patting Iona's cheek with his paw until she woke up and gave him another one. When Iona's parents began sleep coaching her, they taught Iona to give Tigger his dinner right before she went to bed and to give him cat treats only in the daytime (and never in her room!).

Items to Add

First, if there is anything you have been intending to do to your child's room (such as purchasing a better-quality pillow or buying a bigger bed if he or she is about to outgrow the current one), this is an excellent time to make these changes. However, do not feel you *have* to make any major changes such as repainting the room or buying all new furniture. Most of the time, the five-step plan in this book, all by itself, will help your child become a better sleeper. In other words, the issue with your child's poor sleep almost never has to do with the comfort or size of the mattress or the color of the room.

Bedtime Buddy

A Bedtime Buddy (also known as a *security object*) such as a teddy bear, doll, or special blanket is highly recommended as part of your child's new routine.

If your child does not already have a security object, ask your child to pick out a cute stuffed animal from his or her collection (or, you can even take your child shopping for a new one) and begin including this animal in the routine each night. Let's say your child loves to play with his or her giraffe, Giselle. From now on, try to include Giselle in each part of your child's bedtime routine. Giselle can sit on the table near your child during the bedtime snack. Later, Giselle can sit on the edge of the bathtub during bath time and then on the bathroom counter during toothbrushing. Giselle can listen to the bedtime story and be tucked in with your child when you are ready to leave.

This familiar and beloved stuffed animal can help your child feel more relaxed and comfortable in bed by staying behind when you leave at the end of the routine. If you lie down with your child at night, you can also begin putting Giselle between the two of you. A security object can be taken along when your child sleeps elsewhere, such as at a relative's home.

Bedtime Basket

The Bedtime Basket is a small basket containing a book or two (or a quiet toy or two) that your child can use to read or play with in bed until he or she is drowsy enough to fall asleep on his or her own; we will talk much more about this in Chapter 6. In addition to books, this basket could have, for example, a couple of dolls or action figures, a puzzle, a small car, or a drawing pad and pencils. Make sure these are things that aren't *too* interesting, though! The goal is for your child to play with something from the basket while becoming drowsy but to also fall asleep fairly quickly. In the same way you read yourself to sleep, your child will play or read to get drowsy enough to fall asleep. As noted earlier in this chapter when we were talking about reading lights, children who read as part of their bedtime routine are likely to get much more sleep!

Bedtime Tickets

Remember when we talked in Chapter 2 about those callbacks and curtain calls that all kids like to make to put off falling asleep? Bedtime Tickets are a great solution to keep these to a minimum. Bedtime Tickets are small, homemade cards that can be used for one or two small requests once the bedtime routine is over for the next five minutes. They can be traded for any request that requires only *a minute or less* to fulfill (such as retrieving a toy from another room, refilling the water cup on the bedside table, giving a brief back rub, or providing one more escorted trip to the bathroom). You and your child can either create fun and colorful Bedtime Tickets together (by decorating index cards, construction paper, or cardboard with paint, markers, or stickers) or you can copy the ones provided at the back of this book. You will give your child one or two each night. Unused Bedtime Tickets can be redeemed in the morning for a small reward. We will talk about Bedtime Tickets in much more detail in Chapter 7.

Nightlight

Your child's room should have a simple nightlight that stays on all night to provide some soft lighting in the bedroom so that you and your child will be safe when moving around the room at bedtime and any time of night. Nightlights also help your children feel oriented when they wake up during the night.

Reading Light

Be sure your child has a small reading light that he or she can turn off independently. There are so many great options for this: a small headlamp on an adjustable headband, a light that clips onto a book or headboard, or a bedside lamp. This reading light should have a low wattage bulb that is just bright enough to read by but dim enough to make your child's room still feel like it is nighttime. Reading lights are important because children who get more sleep are more likely to read as part of their bedtime routine.*

Important note: Please remember the overhead light in your child's room should be off at night. Your child may like bright lighting when falling asleep, but if you turn this light off later when you go to bed, your child's room will look completely different when he or she awakens during the night (as all children do). Your child will have had no practice falling asleep in this dimmer and darker environment and will want the light on again.

Remember, your child can learn over time to feel comfortable about falling asleep in a room with only a nightlight and small reading light. If you have a child who slips out of bed to turn on the overhead light after you've left the room, you may even need to temporarily remove the bulb from the overhead light (or gradually reduce the wattage of the bulb in the overhead light every few days).

---

*"2004 Sleep in America Poll," National Sleep Foundation (Washington, DC: 2004).

Other Things to Consider Adding

Water. Place a cup of water or water bottle on the bedside table.

Sound machines. Consider what you want to do about sound machines (also known as white noise machines). Many people begin using these in the nursery when their child is an infant, and these are acceptable as long as they stay on all night.

Remember, however, these machines can become another item your child will eventually *need* in order to fall asleep. If you want your child to be able to fall asleep anywhere (at a hotel, a summer camp, a sleepover party, a field trip, or a relative's home), consider *eventually* teaching your child to fall asleep without a sound machine. Since a sound machine is unlikely to be available in these other settings, your child will either have to fall asleep without it or your child may want or need to take it along. (However, if you live in a loud environment such as an apartment building in an urban area, a sound machine may be a useful addition to your child's room.)

Body pillow. Not every child will need this but some may. We will talk more about this in Chapter 6.

Weighted blankets. If your child already likes to use a weighted blanket, be sure you teach him or her to pull this blanket up independently and make sure you won't mind taking it wherever your child goes. These blankets help some children feel safe and relaxed, but they can also be hot, hard to transport, and heavy (not to mention expensive to take along if you are traveling by air).

Some children prefer a weighted blanket alternative such as a stretchy bed wrap. These are pulled up over the bottom of the bed to encircle your child's mattress like a large, tight sock. They provide deep pressure with compression rather than with weight, and they are light, washable, and easy to pack. Most children don't need these types of blankets or bed wraps at all, however, and can learn to sleep well with basic bedding.

Flashlight. Consider adding a small flashlight to your child's room so that he or she can use this to illuminate any part of their room; these are optional, of course, but many kids love them. Keychain flashlights are a great type to consider. These turn on when they are squeezed and then turn off automatically when a child lets go of them when he or she drifts off to sleep. (These may not be the best idea for siblings that share a room, though!)

Timer. Consider having a timer available. Timers can be helpful to mark the end of reading time or to help move your child along if he or she tends to stall or dawdle during any part of the bedtime routine. We will talk more about timers in Chapter 5.

Blackout curtains can sometimes be useful if your child wakes too early or if you want to encourage daytime naps, but these are optional.

A **motion sensor** is not necessary unless it would be useful for you to know your child has left his or her room. For example, if your child has a habit of leaving his or her bedroom and slipping into your bed later without you noticing, you could consider a motion sensor (see Chapter 8). However, if your child sleepwalks, a motion sensor is **strongly recommended**. The motion sensor will beep to alert you that your child is "on the move" anytime he or she leaves the bedroom.

• • •

Before we wrap up this chapter and review the checklist, there are two more useful guidelines you might want to keep in mind.

The Summer Camp Rule

The summer camp rule may help clarify why "simple is best" when you are preparing your child's bedroom for sleep coaching. If you help your child learn to fall asleep with items that he or she could easily take to summer camp, your child will become a confident sleeper who can fall asleep anywhere, whether that might be camp, a new hotel, or a relative's home. For example, a child could easily take a headband-style reading light, a book, a flashlight, and a special blanket to summer camp but would never show up for camp with an essential oil diffuser, a star projector, or a TV!

The 2 a.m. Rule

Once you have removed and added the items above, take a final look around: Will your child's room look, sound, and feel the same at bedtime as it will when your child wakes up in the middle of the night at 2 a.m. (or at whatever time your child often wakes)? If so, this may help your child fall back to sleep much more easily during the night.

WORKSHEET FOR STEP 1

Prepare Your
Child's Bedroom for Great Sleep

Items to Remove from the Bedroom:

___ Electronics

___ Anything that turns off later

___ Pets

Items to Add to the Bedroom:

___ Bedtime Buddy

___ Bedtime Basket

___ Bedtime Tickets

___ Reading light

___ Nightlight

Take a Final Look Around . . .

___ Do the items that your child uses to fall asleep pass the summer camp rule?

___ Will your child's bedroom look the same at 2 a.m. as it does at bedtime?

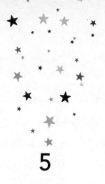

5

STEP 2:
Use the 5B Bedtime Routine
Every Night

Five-year-old James never wanted to go to his bedroom at bedtime. His parents had not really developed a bedtime routine, so James fell asleep on the living room sofa while they watched their favorite shows on TV every night. If they tried to send him up to bed, he told them that he didn't like to be upstairs when they were downstairs and that his room had a "scary window." Every night right after dinner, he brought his pillow and favorite blanket down to the living room couch while his parents did the dishes and then fell asleep there while his parents watched their shows. Once he was deeply asleep, his dad carried him up to bed. Sometimes his parents would hear his footsteps on the stairs in the middle of the night as he was on his way back to the living room to turn the TV back on again. They were sometimes able to intercept him before he made it to the living room and would walk him back to bed. More often, however, they would find him asleep on the living room couch in the morning with the TV on.

James did not really have a consistent bedtime routine to help him become drowsy and comfortable in his bedroom, so he had learned to fall asleep easily only by being near his parents on the living room sofa with the TV on. A child without a regular bedtime routine who learns to fall asleep in another part of the house and who is moved to his bed later only after falling asleep will often report that there is something scary about his room or protest being alone there. However, your child can learn how to settle into sleep quickly, easily, and independently if you use a proven bedtime routine consistently every night that concludes in your child's room.

A well-planned bedtime routine accomplishes the following things:

- it helps your child fall asleep more quickly each night by allowing him or her to feel settled and drowsy,

- it eventually "programs" or cues relaxation and drowsiness if the steps are done in the same order each night,

- it helps avoid stalling and arguments at bedtime, and

- it helps discourage lots of callbacks and curtain calls by including all the things your child really needs.

The 5B Bedtime Routine has five steps that all start with "B" so you and your child can remember the routine more easily. It was designed to be enjoyable and relaxing for both you and your child and should not require more than thirty to forty minutes or so.

It is always good to prepare for any new routine by first discussing it with your child. When it is time to talk about it, you'll want to keep the following in mind:

- Try not to argue about it or defend it.

- Try not to answer endless questions about it.

- Try not to pay much attention to any negative comments about it.

- Try not to talk about it at all once bedtime arrives. Just follow the routine confidently and consistently each night.

Here is a sample script that you could modify for your own child to prepare him or her for the new routine.

Our family is going to use a special bedtime routine for you every night to help you learn how to fall asleep on your own and how to sleep in your own bed all night long. We will be nearby, of course, while you are learning to do this. When our new bedtime routine is over tonight, I am going to give you two Bedtime Tickets. You can use a Bedtime Ticket if you want to get one more thing or to make one more trip out of the room.

After your two Bedtime Tickets are gone, you will need to stay in your bed with your Bedtime Buddy and use the books and toys in your Bedtime Basket until you are drowsy and ready to fall asleep on your own. If you decide not to use one or both of your Bedtime Tickets, you can trade these unused Bedtime Tickets in the morning for a reward!

Make a Personalized
5B Bedtime Routine Chart for Your Child

A 5B Bedtime Routine chart will keep both you and your children on track and will make things go much more smoothly if someone else needs to put your child to bed (a babysitter or a grandparent, for example).

A chart also keeps the routine very consistent from night to night and reduces stalling, complaining, refusals, crying, and delayed reports of being hungry. It's harder to argue with a chart than with a parent! If your child engages in any of these behaviors, refer to the chart and say, "The chart says it's time to . . . (have your bedtime snack, take a bath, brush teeth, and so on)." Then move forward with that step gently but firmly. You may need to offer a "one or the other choice" at times. For example, you may need to say, "Do you want to get out of the bathtub by yourself? Or would you like me to lift you out?" or "Do you want to put on your purple pajamas now? Or your yellow ones?" Either way, keep things moving along from one step to the next, even if you have to offer calm but confident assistance.

You can copy the sample 5B Bedtime Routine Chart, which is in Appendix C at the end of this book, or make your own. To make your own chart, you and your child could find pictures that represent each step of the 5B Bedtime Routine, or you could take your own photographs of your child doing each step and then print these out for the chart. Be sure to add one last picture that shows your child in bed relaxing independently with the Bedtime Buddy and the Bedtime Basket after the 5B Bedtime Routine is over.

Choose a Bedtime and Stick to It!

If you do not choose a specific time to start the routine each night, this will become a negotiation with your child night after night (and surely you don't want that!). It's also essential to turn off all electronics before you begin the 5B Bedtime Routine. Some families like to dim the lights in their home as well to signal the beginning of a quieter and calmer time of the day that is focused on relaxation and rest.

The 5 Bs in the 5B Bedtime Routine

● **Bedtime Bite.** Serve your child a healthy snack and make sure this is eaten only in the kitchen so your child will not associate her bedroom with food. Snacks low in sugar that have some complex carbohydrates and some protein are great choices (for example, nut butter on whole wheat toast).

Serving a substantial snack at the beginning of the routine ensures that your child will not be able to stall the bedtime routine later by telling you he or she is hungry. This will also discourage your child from getting up to eat once you are fast asleep (more children do this than you would think). A substantial bedtime snack might even keep your child from waking too early, and that is often a welcome outcome!

Once snack time is over, teach your child that the kitchen is *closed*. You might even want to send this message by turning off the kitchen lights, closing the kitchen door, and so on, if necessary.

● **Bath.** If it is a bath night, or even if it's not, do some washing up and then your child can change into pajamas.

● **Brushing teeth.**

● **Bathroom.** Provide one last opportunity to go to the bathroom. This may also help avoid extra bathroom requests later.

● **Books.** Read in your child's bed with your child and your child's Bedtime Buddy. A timer can be used to mark the end of reading time or you can choose a very specific number of books to read instead.

Let's talk more about the advantages of using a timer to mark the end of reading time, and more importantly, to mark the *end* of the entire 5B Bedtime Routine:

- A timer ensures that there is no confusion or argument about when the 5B Bedtime Routine is over by clearly marking the end of both reading time and the routine itself when it chimes.

- Timers can be useful when you are putting more than one child to bed. You can set a timer for the amount of time you plan to spend reading with each child. When the timer chimes, you will have a fair and graceful way to make your exit.

- Remember that timers can also be used for *any other specific part* of the routine to help move your child along if he or she tends to stall or dawdle. During snack time, for example, you could use the timer to allot a certain amount of time to eat the bedtime snack, or you could set a timer for the amount of time you'd like your child to be in the bathtub.

Important note: Before the final step in the 5B Bedtime Routine (in other words, before the Books step), feel free to add any other step your child has become accustomed to at bedtime. For example, if you always sing a special song or always give your child a special kind of foot rub, add this step just before Books (and add this step to the Bedtime Routine Chart, too!). Just remember two things. Any step you add to the routine should not require leaving the bedroom and should not be overly physical. For example, any wrestling, hide and seek, dance-offs, and so on, should happen *before* the 5B Bedtime Routine is begun.

The bedtime routine must *always* conclude in your child's room so that your child learns to fall asleep in her own bed each night. If you fell asleep in your bed in the master bedroom and woke up somewhere else later, you would be disoriented and would likely want to return to the place where you fell asleep.

Finally, be very sure your child does not fall asleep during *any part* of the 5B Bedtime Routine. Your goal is for your child to fall asleep on his or her own *after* the

5B Bedtime Routine is over by self-comforting! You will be present, at first, while he or she does this, but your child will need to learn to self-comfort when you two are not interacting. You will review exactly how to do this in the next chapter.

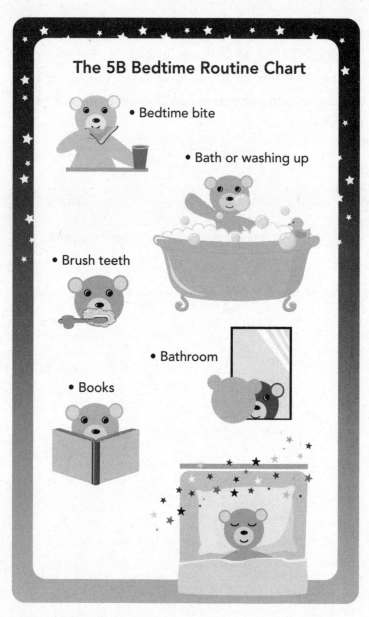

The 5B Bedtime Routine Chart

• Bedtime bite

• Bath or washing up

• Brush teeth

• Bathroom

• Books

(A printable *5B Bedtime Routine Chart* is on page 220.)

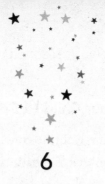

6

STEP 3:
Teach Your Child to Self-Comfort
as You Work Your Way Out

Nine-year-old Levi really, really wanted to go to camp with his friends during the upcoming summer. January, February, and March came and went, and his family still had not sent in the deposit and paperwork. This was because both Levi and his parents were worried that he would not be able to sleep well at camp because he had such a hard time falling asleep each night. Even in his own home, he always needed one of his parents to sit in a beanbag chair in his room until he was deeply asleep. His room was dim at bedtime, and it was hard to see the beanbag chair, so he often sat up and checked to make sure that a parent was still in the chair. Each night, it took Levi more than two hours to fall asleep.

Teach Your Child to Self-Comfort

After the 5B Bedtime Routine concludes, it's important to send a clear message that the bedtime routine is now over and it is time for your child to learn how to put himself or herself to sleep independently. Turn off any overhead lights or room lamps and leave on only the nightlight and the reading light. Give your child a final hug and kiss, and tuck him or her into bed with the Bedtime Buddy and Bedtime Basket. Remind your child to snuggle the Bedtime Buddy and read or play quietly and independently with items from the Bedtime Basket until drowsy enough to fall asleep on his or her own.

Remember, your child should have only water to drink, should not be listening to any music, should not have access to any electronics, should not be given any type of blanket tuck that only you can do "the right way," and should not have the family pet on the bed.

Once your child is reading or playing quietly in bed, try not to worry about how long it takes your child to become drowsy and fall asleep. As a matter of fact, initially your child is likely to be awake for *longer* than usual since he or she is just learning this new skill of self-comforting. So, calmly and lovingly give your child the space he or she needs, as long as he or she stays in bed playing or reading quietly.

Remember when your child was a baby and your pediatrician advised you to put your child into the crib when he or she was *drowsy but awake* so that your child would learn to self-comfort? This is exactly what your older child is now learning how to do.

Since your child has the Bedtime Buddy and the Bedtime Basket, he or she no longer has to lie in bed awake (and perhaps anxious or upset!) in the dark. Your child can instead relax and play quietly with the Bedtime Buddy and read or play with items from the Bedtime Basket. Your child will learn to relax quietly until he or she is drowsy, just as you probably do. If you feel concerned about how long it takes your child to read himself or herself to sleep, remember that it probably already takes your child a long time to fall asleep now. Also, being able to self-comfort to sleep at bedtime will soon lead to fewer and shorter wakings during the night. Your child will get better at this over time and this is a skill your child can use for life!

Once your child is reading or playing, you are "off duty" and can begin the process of tapering your presence gradually while engaging in your own activities.

Work Your Way Out of the Room

Four-year-old Bella had become used to falling asleep each night by playing with her mother's curly hair while her mother rubbed Bella's tummy and they sang the "ABC" song over and over. It took Bella more than an hour to fall asleep every night (and many, many rounds of the "ABC" song). Bella refused to settle down at night at all if her father tried to do the bedtime routine. Bella's mother and father had not been out on a date since Bella had turned three and her parents missed their time together as a couple.

Bella's mother knew she had to change the way she put Bella to bed. First, she changed their bedtime routine so that they sang the "ABC" song together only once while Bella's mother gave Bella a tummy rub. They read two books together as the last step in their bedtime routine.

Next, since Bella loved ponies, her mom bought her a small stuffed pony with a curly mane. Bella named this pony Piper, and Piper became her favorite Bedtime Buddy. Bella learned to fall asleep playing with Piper's mane every night while her mother sat in a chair nearby. Soon, Bella's dad could put Bella to sleep since she no longer needed to play with her mother's hair. Once Bella's parents could alternate putting her to sleep, they knew that she would soon be able to fall asleep for her grandmother, which would allow them to have a date night every week or so.

If you have been comforting your child to sleep by being very nearby, you will now learn how to gradually reduce the amount of comforting you are providing. While you are doing this, your child will be using the Bedtime Buddy and Bedtime Basket to practice self-comforting. If you want your child to be a great sleeper, you will definitely want to help your child learn to fall asleep without having you nearby.

Children who need you to comfort them to sleep at bedtime often take much longer to fall asleep. This is because they worry that you might leave before the job is done or because you might not provide this comfort in the exact same way each night. This can happen because you might not have the same amount of patience on one night as you do on another! Children are also often unable to return to sleep after awakening at night because when you leave, your comforting behaviors leave, too.

Let's first identify all of the most common comforting behaviors you might be using at bedtime now so that you will be sure to recognize everything your child is currently depending on. Comforting behaviors that are provided by a parent, as we reviewed in Chapter 2, are often called "sleep crutches" or "sleep props." Don't worry, your child *can* learn to fall asleep without the sleep crutches you currently provide, but the first step is to use this checklist to identify which ones you are currently using:

___ Lying in bed with your child (or staying *very* nearby, perhaps at the bottom of the bed or in a chair near the bed)

___ Allowing your child to touch you in a very specific way in order to fall asleep. For example, some children like to twirl a lock of their parent's hair, rub a parent's earlobe or cheek, wrap an arm or a leg over a parent, touch their parent's feet with their feet, put their head on their parent's shoulder, lie very close to their parent's side, or hold their parent's hand.

___ Touching your child in a very specific way to help your child fall asleep. For example, you might be rubbing your child's back or head. You might be wrapping one or both arms around your child. You might be combing through your child's hair with your fingers.

___ Singing or talking for long periods to your child.

___ Reading books or telling long stories to your child until he or she falls asleep.

Behaviors on the list above *do not* cause a problem if they occur during the bedtime routine *well before* your child is ready to fall asleep, but are problematic if they are happening *as your child is actually falling asleep.*

Once you have identified all of the things you are currently providing, you will need to stop offering these when the bedtime routine is over and allow your child to learn to self-comfort with the Bedtime Buddy and items in the

Bedtime Basket. You will need to offer only your presence in your child's bed or in a chair next to the bed while your child is learning this skill.

Have you been staying with your child for years to help him or her fall asleep? Remember, you will need to work your way out of the room *very gradually* at bedtime if you have been staying with your child for a long period of time to help him or her fall asleep. *Anything else will be too difficult and abrupt for your child.* This book was written because these behaviors are very common, so leave behind any guilt you may have and know that your child will soon be a wonderful, independent sleeper! You will gradually move farther and farther away over the course of a few days or weeks while your child practices self-comforting.

There is one very important thing to keep in mind when you begin the process of tapering your presence: **your child will protest this and is likely to express frustration with you!** Your child's behavior at bedtime is also likely to get even worse for a few nights. This is normal. You are asking your child to change how he or she falls asleep, and your child is comfortable with the old way. Keep in mind that if you had to learn to fall asleep with a strange new type of pillow, for example, you would be likely to protest, too. Try to project calm confidence in your child's ability to learn this new way to fall asleep. Be kind but firm and stick to the plan. This is a very gradual and gentle plan, and, with time and patience, your child can definitely learn this new method.

If your child wants to have long discussions about why you will no longer be providing so much assistance (patting, cuddling, and so on) at bedtime, you can avoid this by simply stating what you *are* going to provide. You might say something like, "I'm going to stay right here in your bed with you, but I'm not going to put my arm around you anymore while you are falling asleep."

If your child continues to protest about this change, you can say something like, "I can only stay here in your bed if we lie side by side without my arm around you." If your child protests for a very long period of time or in a way that becomes problematic (for example, by yelling at you), you can get up and stand next to the bed, repeat a simple sentence like the one above but with a phrase about the behavior you do not want, and then return to the bed again. For example, you might use a phrase like, "If you yell at me, you are telling me that you do not want me in your bed. I can only stay here in your bed if we lie quietly side by side."

You may need to repeat this sequence by getting out of bed a few times if you have a very determined child, but remember, your child *wants you nearby.* He or she will agree to this new arrangement fairly quickly if you are calm, confident, and firm, and if you remove your presence briefly and then return. These gentle changes are not harmful to your child in any way because you are providing your calm presence throughout this process. In fact, soon your child (and probably everyone else in your family) will be getting more sleep, which benefits all of you. You will need to decide how to begin based on what your child is used to. The steps below assume that your child has a "preferred parent" (which is not uncommon, of course!) who has been lying or sitting in the child's bed most of the time. If this is not true for your family, just begin on the step below that matches what your child is currently used to. If there is a preferred parent, this parent will work on the first step, and then parents should begin alternating every other night or so once there is a body pillow between you and your child (see below).

- Sit or lie in your child's bed silently after reading time is over and allow your child to read or play in bed until he or she falls asleep. You can act like you are asleep, or as long as you keep the lighting soft, you can read, listen to a podcast or audio book, or do some work. *Be sure not to give in and provide the sleep crutches that involve touch if your child stays awake for a long time.* Just provide your silent presence.

- Once your child can fall asleep easily with just your silent presence in the bed, put a long body pillow (or rolled-up quilt or blanket) between you and your child. Once you put the body pillow in place, begin alternating parents from now on. One night could be Mom's night and the next could be Dad's, for example, or whatever schedule works for your family. If your child prefers one parent or caregiver over another, be sure you do not allow the preferred parent to come in *later* to provide some final comforting. For example, if it's Dad's night, and your child prefers Mom, let your child know that you are serious about alternating parents by saying something like, "It's Dad's night or no one's night. Mom is not coming in later."

Allow your child to read or play in bed until he or she falls asleep. You can either act like you are asleep or, as long as you keep the lighting soft, you can read, listen to a podcast or audio book with an earphone, or do some work. *Be sure not to give in and provide the sleep crutches that involve touch if your child is awake for a long time.* Just provide your silent presence.

- Once your child can fall asleep easily with a body pillow between the two of you, move to a chair right next to your child's bed and leave the body pillow behind for your child. Allow your child to read or play in bed until he or she falls asleep. You can act like you are asleep while you are in the chair, or as long as you keep the lighting soft, you can read, listen to a podcast or audio book, or do some work.

Important note: Once you have reached this step, **do not sit or lie in your child's bed anymore to help him or her fall asleep**. From this point on, you should be in a chair.

- Once your child can fall asleep easily with you in a chair, move the chair halfway to the door. Allow your child to read or play in bed until he or she falls asleep. You can act like you are asleep while you are in the chair, or as long as you keep the lighting soft, you can read, listen to a podcast or audio book, or do some work.

- Once your child can fall asleep easily with the chair halfway to the door, move the chair to the doorway and face out into the hallway. Allow your child to read or play in bed until he or she falls asleep. You can act like you are asleep while you are in the chair, or as long as you keep the lighting soft, you can read, listen to a podcast or audio book, or do some work.

- Once your child can fall asleep easily with the chair in the doorway, move the chair into the hallway but rustle the pages of your book or your papers, or type softly on your laptop so that he or she can *hear* you but not *see* you. Allow your child to read or play in bed until he or she falls asleep. You can act like you are asleep while you are in the chair, or as long as you keep the lighting soft, you can read, listen to a podcast or audio book, or do some work.

- Once your child can fall asleep easily with you out of sight in the hallway, stay on the same floor. Allow your child to read or play in bed until he or she falls asleep.

- Once your child can fall asleep easily with you on the same floor, you can be anywhere in your home. Allow your child to read or play in bed until he or she falls asleep.

- Once your child can fall asleep easily with you anywhere in the home . . . book the sitter!

Parents often ask how long they should wait before moving on to the next step. Stay on each step until your child can fall asleep quickly and easily on that step, and then move on to the next step. Any resistance your child expresses with regard to the next step is a sign that your child is not yet sure that he or she will know how to fall asleep when you are in the new spot. However, this is a gradual plan and one that builds your child's confidence by helping him or her make progress slowly but consistently.

Stick with the plan and remind your child that he or she has already achieved success with the earlier steps. Express your confidence in your child and move in a matter-of-fact way to your new spot once your child can fall asleep easily on the prior step. Remember that it may take your child a bit longer to get himself or herself to sleep after you move to the new step. Just let your child read or play as you always do, and he or she will soon be successful. Once your child is deeply asleep, you may leave the room or floor. If your child wakes up again before it is time for you to go to bed, return to the step you were using at bedtime (for example, sitting in a chair near the bed with a body pillow in bed with your child).

Don't forget to alternate nights with your spouse, partner or other caregiver, and try not to ever move *backward* once your child has progressed to the next step. Once your child can fall asleep independently, you will feel much more comfortable about leaving home in the evening for a date with your partner or spouse, an outing with a friend, or any other event. This process might take *weeks*, but remember that this issue might have been months or years in the making!

It can be really helpful to make a list with each step so that your child can see what the next step will be and will know what to expect. This also heads off any attempts by your child to bargain or to try to change the plan.

WORKSHEET FOR STEP 3

Work Your Way Out of the Room with the Following Steps:

1. Parent in bed with child

2. Parent in bed with child with body pillow between child and parent

3. Parent in chair near the bed while body pillow remains in bed with child

4. Parent in chair halfway to the door

5. Parent in chair in the doorway facing out

6. Parent in chair in hallway

7. Parent is on the same floor as child

8. Parent is anywhere in the home

Once your child can fall asleep easily with a parent anywhere in the home ... book the sitter!

7

STEP 4:
Limit Callbacks and Curtain Calls

Five-year-old Ria liked to make at least a dozen callbacks and curtain calls every night for "just one more" thing. Once her mother introduced the concept of Bedtime Tickets, Ria used one bedtime ticket at night and saved one to trade for her favorite reward each morning: doing an art project with her mother.

While your child is learning to self-comfort and you are working your way out of the room, your child is also very likely to try to interact with you by using callbacks and curtain calls instead of getting down to the business of learning how to relax into sleep on his or her own. There are several ways to manage this often-difficult time of the evening. Let's start with Bedtime Tickets since these will be the first line of defense!

Use Bedtime Tickets

You can let your child know that if she needs anything else from you while she is learning to self-comfort, she can use a Bedtime Ticket. You've already learned in Chapter 2 (How Do Sleep Problems Get Started in the First Place?) that you may actually have been rewarding your child for staying awake by allowing her to call you back for many more requests or by allowing her to come out of her bedroom many times after the bedtime routine has concluded.

You allow these behaviors, of course, because you hope that once you have granted all of these requests, your child will finally fall asleep. This never turns out to be true because, in actuality, calling you back for more books and backrubs and conversations is *waaay* more fun than getting down to the business of falling asleep, and responding to all of these requests keeps your child awake longer!

Bedtime Tickets are the answer to this issue. Use the ones you created in Chapter 4 or make copies of the sample Bedtime Tickets provided in Appendix C. Give your child one or two tickets at the end of the 5B Bedtime Routine. Your child can use these during the next five minutes for one or two *brief* requests or trips out of the room. These requests should take only *one minute or less*. For example, your child might want one more hug or one last trip to the bathroom. These tickets *expire* after five minutes.

Bedtime Tickets are very useful because they provide a sense of control for both parents and children:

- Parents may be aware that they grant too many requests after lights out, but they often do not have a simple way to manage this problem. Bedtime Tickets allow parents to feel good about setting limits while still knowing that their children can request one or two more things, if necessary.

- Children learn how to recognize when the bedtime routine is over while still being allowed one or two more brief interactions with a parent. Tickets allow your child to feel that he or she has some control over the bedtime process but not so much control that the bedtime routine continues indefinitely.

Tickets help to give the bedtime routine a clear endpoint. Your child can then get on with the process of learning how to fall asleep independently. A bedtime routine *without* a clear endpoint results in stalling, lost sleep time, sleep-deprived kids, and exhausted and frustrated parents.

Once children learn that their parents grant only one or two more requests when the bedtime routine is over, they settle into sleep more quickly because they know that when the tickets are gone, they will not miss out on any additional parental attention.

Children learn that they *can* use a Bedtime Ticket to see you once more, but they don't *have* to. This is similar to how you, as an adult, might feel if you had a mild over-the-counter sleeping pill in the medicine cabinet. You wouldn't use it every night, but you might be glad to have it on hand if needed.

Parents and children will eventually sleep better and with fewer sleep disruptions during the night, since children who fall asleep without so many parental interactions at bedtime can return to sleep on their own more easily when they awaken at night.

• • •

Let's summarize how to use Bedtime Tickets:

- Your child will be given one or two tickets at the end of the 5B Bedtime Routine.

- Each ticket is good for one brief request.

- Bedtime Tickets expire in five minutes.

- Unused tickets can be redeemed the next morning for a small reward (see chart on the next page).

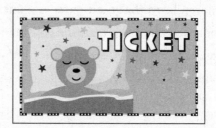

BEDTIME TICKET REWARDS

Unused Bedtime Tickets can be redeemed in the morning for a reward. Your child probably already has some favorite rewards, but the following list may give you some new ideas.

- Choosing a small toy from a grab bag or unwrapping an inexpensive "mystery" gift. (Discount or party stores often have small, inexpensive toys.)
- Getting a sticker
- Making a craft item or baking a treat
- Going to get ice cream
- Choosing a special breakfast treat, after school snack, or lunch bag item
- Having a friend over for a special type of play date
- Getting an extra book at reading time
- Skipping one small daily chore
- Going on a special outing (the skate park, the movies, a hiking trail)
- Having an indoor or outdoor picnic
- Getting a new book from the library

Weekly rewards (for redeeming five to seven Bedtime Tickets) might be:

- Getting some new supplies for a favorite hobby
- Having a sleepover
- Doing a larger baking or cooking project
- Doing a more involved craft or science project
- Buying a new book or a new toy

Once the Bedtime Tickets are used or have expired, try to minimize talking and avoid granting further requests by using the following techniques.

Be Quiet . . . Be Very, Very Quiet!

Eight-year-old Liliana became very chatty about her friends and her school day once the bedtime routine was over and it was time for her to read or play on her own until she was drowsy enough to fall asleep. Her mother liked chatting with her about these things during that part of the routine because she, of course, loved hearing more about what Liliana was thinking and feeling. However, Liliana's mother worried that these long bedtime talks were leading to some loss of sleep for Liliana, and she wanted to find another time when Liliana could chat with her about her day.

Many kids will tell you that nothing happened at school that day on the car ride home, but those same kids will become chatterboxes full of fascinating information once it's time for them to get down to the business of falling asleep. If this scenario fits your child, try to find another time during the evening to have this kind of talk with your child. Maybe you two could talk in a cozy corner of the kitchen while having hot cocoa and the bedtime snack, for example.

However, once the bedtime routine is over, try not to have deep talks with your child about his or her innermost feelings. Why? Because this could worsen your child's sleep in two ways:

- Your child may become much more talkative around bedtime to ensure that you stay nearby for long periods of time.

- Your child may talk with you about something that was upsetting that day, such as an experience that made your child angry or anxious. This might lead to your child's bed being associated with negative feelings. Ideally, your child's bed should be associated only with relaxation and sleep. Try to find another time and place to have this kind of talk with your child.

If there is one secret to moving things along quickly while you are helping your child learn to self-comfort and fall asleep quickly, it is this: *be present while your child is learning to self-soothe—but be as silent as possible.* You will be nearby, of course, as you help your child learn this new sleep skill, but try very hard to be silent.

Try not to do anything else while your child plays or reads until drowsy enough to fall asleep. *Your child has already had lots of special time with you during the 5B Bedtime Routine,* plus one or two more interactions if he or she used the Bedtime Tickets.

By keeping any further interaction with your child brief and boring, you are teaching your child that you are serious about the bedtime routine being over and about helping him or her learn this new skill of falling asleep independently. Your child will soon learn that you are not going to give in or change your mind.

Your silent presence helps your child master the skills necessary to fall asleep independently much more rapidly because he will learn that you won't be interacting with him at all even though you are still nearby.

Repeat a "Broken Record" Phrase

Five-year-old Zoe did not like it when her father stayed silent after the bedtime routine was over. At first, while she was learning to fall asleep independently, she had plenty more to say: "You're not fun at bedtime anymore, Dad!" or "I'm so bored!" or "I'm not sleepy" or even "I'm lonely!" (even though her dad was sitting right next to her bed).

As noted before, your child will protest this new routine at first. Remember that your silent presence during this process is best, but if it is just too difficult for you not to respond at all when your child talks to you, then quietly and calmly repeat the same phrase each time: **"Your Bedtime Tickets are gone. Read or play until you are sleepy. It's**

bedtime." Don't get drawn into a discussion or let your feelings get hurt from one of your child's complaints. (After all, you don't get upset when your children complain about your parenting when you don't let them eat brownies before dinner!) Each and every time your child talks or calls out to you, repeat this same, exact phrase until your child is asleep. This is called the "broken record" technique and is meant to show your child that nothing else interesting is going to happen. Things are going to be really boring from this point on. Your child may as well give up on stalling and fall asleep!

Handle Extra Bathroom Requests

Your child can use a Bedtime Ticket for an "escorted trip" to the bathroom if he or she has one left. Otherwise, if your child asks to go the bathroom again after the Bedtime Tickets have been used or have expired, ask him or her to go independently. You can use a timer if your child seems to be stalling once in the bathroom, if need be.

If your child requests many trips to the bathroom, you could try putting a portable potty in your child's room so that he or she does not have to leave the room. This is also useful if your child calls you back frequently at bedtime to take him or her to the bathroom once you no longer need to stay in the room after the bedtime routine ends. Most children become a lot less interested in going to the bathroom if they don't get an escorted trip from mom and dad.

Move to a Chair in the Doorway

Six-year-old Darius did not like the new bedtime routine at all at first and would test the limits of the new routine by laughing, jumping out of the bed, running out of the room, and hiding in other parts of the house when the routine was over. Bedtime tickets did not work, either. He would quickly use both of them and then still bolt out of the room over and over again. His parents had to keep bringing him back, and they were losing their patience.

Sometimes, while you are working your way through this process, your child may really test your limits. He may do this even while you are still on one of the steps that keeps you very nearby. If your child becomes very disruptive by yelling at you, leaving the bed multiple times, or running out of the room, for example, you may need to use an interim step.

If your child chooses any of these more disruptive behaviors, move out of the bed and sit in a chair in the doorway. (If you were already in a chair near your child's bed, just move this chair to the doorway.) Sit with your back to your child's room and remind your child that you will move back to where you were only when he stays in bed and reads or plays quietly while getting drowsy enough to fall asleep.

Be very quiet while you are in the doorway. Pay no attention to requests, questions, or attempts at conversation, and make sure your child cannot leave the room. You may need a very wide chair (or even a gate) if your child tests you by trying to slip out. If you choose to use a gate, put your chair just outside the gate.

Some children will make getting out of bed into a game. If so, help your child back to bed no more than twice. After that, don't keep putting your child back to bed. Just sit in the doorway with your back to the room. Wait quietly without talking until your child falls asleep, no matter where that might be (on a rug in his room, in his beanbag chair, or wherever). Once your child is deeply asleep, you can move him or her back to the bed.

Remember, even though your child is protesting this new way of falling asleep, having your calm, physical presence in the doorway lets your child know he or she is safe.

Use Calm, Silent Walk Backs

Mateo had learned to fall asleep quickly and independently, but after a month or so he began coming out into the living room again many times to ask his parents lots of questions instead reading himself to sleep.

Once you no longer need to be present in your child's room when the bedtime routine is over, walk your child back to his room calmly and silently *each and every time* he leaves the room. You can also say the broken record phrase again, if you wish (**"Your Bedtime Tickets are gone. Read or play until you are sleepy. It's bedtime."**). If this becomes a problem every night, just go back to sitting silently in a chair in the doorway with your back to your child's room and make sure your child cannot leave the room.

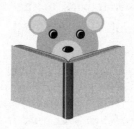

WORKSHEET FOR STEP 4
Limit Callbacks and Curtain Calls

- **Use Bedtime Tickets.** Give your child two tickets for any callbacks and curtain calls. These expire in five minutes and unused ones earn a reward in the morning.

- **Be quiet** . . . be very, very quiet. Or if you feel you need to respond, repeat a broken record phrase: **"Your Bedtime Tickets are gone. Read or play until you are sleepy. It's bedtime."**

- **Handle extra bathroom requests.** Your child can use a Bedtime Ticket for an escorted trip, your child can go independently, or your child can use a portable potty in his or her room.

- If your child acts out loudly or disruptively, **sit in a chair in the doorway with your back to your child,** being very quiet until your child is calmer and in bed again and then go back to the step you were on OR just stay in the chair in the doorway until your child falls asleep.

- **Use calm, silent walk backs** if your child leaves the room for any reason.

8

STEP 5:
Manage Night and
Early Morning Wakings

Six-year-old Emma fell asleep in her own bed each night after the 5B Bedtime Routine, but just after midnight most nights when her parents were deeply asleep, Emma slipped undetected into her parents' bed like a little ninja and stayed until morning. Emma's parents needed a way to manage these nightly visits.

Your child is likely to keep coming to your room at night until she learns how to fall asleep easily at bedtime on her own without you present in the room at all, so let's talk about how to manage night wakings and early morning wakings as you wait for your child to master this skill.

Make a Plan for Night Wakings

Once you have reached the step where you are sitting in a chair when your child falls asleep at bedtime, you can choose from four methods to manage night wakings. (If you are still on a step that requires you to lie in your child's bed at bedtime, just return to your child's bed after a night waking and help your child return to sleep the exact same way you were doing this at bedtime.)

The method you choose to manage night wakings depends on your own parental preferences. When you choose the method you want to use, keep in mind that these wakings *almost always decrease in frequency* once your child can fall asleep independently at bedtime without you in the room. Also, whichever method you choose, keep your interactions with your child brief at night. You want your child's night wakings to be boring, not rewarding or entertaining!

Method One: Set Up a Temporary Spare Bed

Set up a temporary spare bed in your child's room. With this method, you would come to your child's room if he or she calls out to you after an awakening (or you would walk your child back to his or her own room if he or she has come to you) and then you would lie down in this spare bed in your child's room after tucking your child back in to his or her bed. The spare bed could be a sleeping bag, air mattress, or twin mattress that you have placed in that room temporarily.

Once you get into the spare bed, face away from your child and act like you are asleep until your child falls asleep. Pay very little attention to your child as you lie in the spare bed so that he or she practices self-comforting back to sleep. You can remain on the spare bed until morning or move back to your own bed once your child is asleep. If moving back to your bed results in your child waking multiple times during the night, just stay in your child's room in the spare bed. Over time, once your child learns to fall asleep independently at bedtime, these night wakings will decrease. You can also gradually move this spare bed out of your child's bedroom toward the door and then out of the room completely once your child masters the skill of falling asleep independently at bedtime and wakes less at night.

This method is a good one because it teaches your child to *wake up in his or her own room every morning*. This helps a child learn that the shift from feeling anxious after an awakening to feeling relaxed can happen in his or her own room rather than in your room.

Method Two:
Sit in a Chair in Your Child's Room

With this method, you would come to your child's room if he or she calls out to you after an awakening (or you would walk your child back to his or her own room if he or she has come to you) and then you would tuck your child back in to his or her bed and sit in a chair.

Once you sit in the chair, face away from your child and be very quiet. It's also fine to act as though you are asleep until your child falls asleep. Move back to your own bed once your child is asleep. If moving back to your bed results in multiple awakenings, you may need to move back to Method One to avoid losing a lot of sleep yourself.

This method is good because it also teaches your child to *wake up in his or her own room every morning*. It helps a child learn that the shift from feeling anxious after an awakening to feeling relaxed can happen in his or her own room rather than in your room.

Method Three:
Walk Your Child Back to the Bedroom

Once your child is falling asleep independently at bedtime easily and quickly and night wakings are rare, just walk your child back to his or her room every time he or she comes out, give him or her a quick tuck, stay a moment, and then go back to your own room. If you do not walk your child back every single time, he or she will learn that there is a certain time of the night that you will give up on this and let him or her into your room. He or she will then come in again and again until you give in and let him or her stay.

Method Four:
Make a "Nest" in Your Room

You have worked hard to teach your child to fall asleep independently and in his or her own room each night. But sometimes this process is exhausting and some children are more persistent than others. If you want to start with a step that might help you to get more sleep at night, you can set up a temporary "nest" in your room. The nest can be a loveseat, a small spare mattress, a sleeping bag on some couch cushions, or some other type of small bed. When your child comes to your room at night, direct him or her to this nest to go back to sleep. Try practicing this before bedtime, so your child will know where to go. Make sure your child knows that he or she is allowed in your room but not in your bed.

Make sure you also send the message to your child that unless he is quiet after coming in, he or she will be walked back quickly to his or her own room. You might say, for example, "If you come to our room during the night, you will need to come in quietly and go back to sleep in this special bed that's just for you. Otherwise, we will walk you back to your bed." Stick to your guns on this rule from the start, even if it means multiple walk backs at first.

Finally, is your child able to sneak into your bed at night without you knowing or waking? Many kids are able to do so; kids are like little ninjas! If so, you may want to set up a system that allows you to be more aware of your child's arrival in your room. For example, you could install a door latch or a motion sensor on your door (or on your child's), so that you would know right away if your child leaves his or her room to come to yours. If you used a latch or a motion sensor, for example, you would hear your child trying to open the latched door, or you would hear the beep that the motion sensor makes when your child crosses the threshold of his or her room (or yours). You will be able to handle these night wakings before he or she makes it into your bed.

Again, remember that nighttime awakenings tend to decrease significantly once your child learns to fall asleep independently at bedtime. Also remember to keep lights to a minimum during any wakings and be sure to avoid any eating and any drinking at night except for water. Finally, always avoid using any electronics to get your child back to sleep.

Make a Plan for Early Morning Wakings

Antonio, a four-year-old, began waking up each morning at 4:30 a.m. He would come to his parents' room to tell them that he was hungry or ready to play. Antonio's parents had tried many things to encourage him to sleep later but none seemed to work.

If your child wakes up too early each morning, you have some options to improve this as well.

Evaluate What Might Be Waking Your Child

Does your child's room get bright too early? Try blackout curtains.

Does your child wake to use the bathroom? If so, make sure your child always goes to the bathroom after any night or early morning waking. Try not to talk or turn on any lights. Nightlights in the hall and bathroom are fine, of course.

You can also try giving him or her fewer liquids in the hour or two before bed.

Finally, you can try rewarding your child for going to the bathroom independently and then returning to bed.

Does your child wake up hungry? Try either having your child eat dinner later or giving your child a more substantial bedtime snack. The bedtime snack would ideally contain some protein (nut butter on toast, for example). It can actually also be very helpful to hold off on giving your child breakfast until the rise time you would prefer. This will help to set your child's "breakfast clock" to that time each morning.

If none of these options work, you can try leaving a simple snack (a bowl with some dry cereal, for example, and some water) on the bedside table. It's better not to associate your child's room with eating, however.

Do noises wake your child? Perhaps your neighbors leave for work very early or maybe there are construction noises disrupting your child's sleep in the early morning hours. Try white noise machines, floor fans, or other sound-blocking techniques such as soft foam earplugs, thick curtains, or rugs that absorb noise.

Does your child wake up to use electronics? Keep these off limits until a certain time of the morning. Remind your child that he or she can use items in the Bedtime Basket in the morning instead.

Finally, choose a time that your child is allowed to come out of his or her room, and don't provide much attention to your child before this time. Otherwise, early wake-ups will be the rule rather than the exception.

Try the Good Morning Lamp

Priya was a four-year-old who was being raised by her grandmother. Priya came almost silently to her grandmother's bed each morning at 4:45 a.m. and touched her grandmother's cheek, often startling her awake. Priya's grandmother hoped to teach Priya to stay in bed later so she set up a Good Morning Lamp for Priya. She taught Priya that if she played quietly in her bed with her toys and stuffed animals until the Good Morning Lamp came on, she would get a small reward. Priya soon began either sleeping later or playing with her toys until the Good Morning Lamp came on, and then she loved climbing into her grandmother's bed for some extra morning snuggles.

Many families enjoy using the "Good Morning Lamp." Young children often do not have an easy way to tell time and so do not know whether it's still time for sleep or time to get up. The Good Morning Lamp gives them a way to do this and children will often begin sleeping later with this technique.

To use the Good Morning Lamp technique, put a small lamp in your child's room and plug it into a timer. This timer is the kind you would use to turn on and off lights when you are away on vacation, for example, and can be found at any home improvement store.

The timer is set to turn the lamp on when your child is allowed to come out of their room (or into your bed for an early morning cuddle). At first, the timer should be set so that the lamp comes on at about the time the child is currently waking (even if this is much earlier that you would prefer) so that your child will get a quick reward for grasping the idea. If your child tries to get up before the lamp comes on, remind him or her that "if the light is off, it is still bedtime." Within a week, your child should be able to make the connection that the lamp signals the time when she is allowed to leave her room. Then you can begin setting the timer to turn the lamp on about fifteen minutes later each week until you reach the rise time that works well for everyone.

The lamp should be set far enough away from your child's bed so that the click of the lamp coming on will not wake your child if he or she is still sleeping, but close enough your child can see it easily. If your child wakes up before the lamp comes on, she would need to either stay in her room until it does come on (playing with the Bedtime Buddy or items from the Bedtime Basket), or come to your room and go to the nest (as described earlier in this chapter). Once the lamp comes on, your child could snuggle with you in your bed.

You could also use a radio or music player instead of a lamp. You would then tell your child that he or she can leave her room when the music begins playing softly.

With the Good Morning Lamp, your child still has the chance to spend some time cuddling with you in your bed but will not be in your bed most of the night. This technique provides a clear signal about when a trip to your room or bed is allowed. In addition, your sleep will not be interrupted constantly, and your child will learn to go back to sleep independently during the night and in the early morning.

Provide Rewards and
Reinforcement in the Morning

If your child made any progress at all at bedtime, provide lots of praise in the morning. If your child still has one of the Bedtime Tickets left, he or she can trade it in the morning for a reward. Try to provide more rewards early in the process; later, once things are going well, you can begin requiring two Bedtime Tickets for a reward, then three, and so on. You will want to make sure your child likes the rewards, so it can be helpful if your child has some choice about what they will be. Please see Chapter 7 for a list of reward ideas.

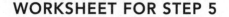

WORKSHEET FOR STEP 5

Manage Night and
Early Morning Awakenings

For *night* wakings, choose from these options:

- Spare bed for a parent in your child's room
- Chair for a parent in the child's doorway
- Walk backs only
- Nest for your child in your room

For *early morning* wakings, use this checklist to address anything that might be waking your child:

- Wakes up due to room brightness?
- Wakes up to use the bathroom?
- Wakes up hungry?
- Wakes up due to noise?
- Wakes up to use electronics?

Remember to provide rewards and reinforcement in the morning!

PART III

Special Concerns

"We are such stuff as dreams are made on;
and our little life is rounded with sleep."
—*William Shakespeare*

Now that you know how to use the five-step guide to help your child become a great sleeper, let's review any special concerns you may have. Chapter 9 will help you determine if your child might have a medical sleep disorder or might benefit from a sleep study. Chapter 10 will help teach you how to sleep coach a child who tends to be more anxious about change or new routines. Chapter 11 will review how to deal with nightmares, night terrors, sleepwalking, and bedwetting. You may want to review Chapter 12 if you have a child on the autism spectrum or one who has behavioral difficulties.

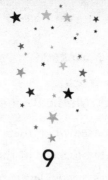

9

Could My Child Have a Medical Sleep Disorder or Need a Sleep Study?

Most children do not have a medical sleep disorder and will never need a sleep study because the vast majority of childhood sleep issues are behavioral and can be resolved with a behavioral plan like the one in this book. But sometimes parents notice something about their child's sleep that concerns them. Perhaps their child seems to gasp or choke at night and they want to rule out a sleep disorder before they begin sleep coaching.

If this is true for you, please review the symptoms of the most common childhood sleep disorders by using the checklist below. If you find any symptoms that do concern you, share these with your child's pediatrician before beginning the five-step plan in this book. It's really important to remember, however, that if your child can fall asleep easily and quickly if you are present and only has difficulty sleeping when you are not, he or she may not have a medical sleep disorder.

Types of Medical Sleep Issues

Sleep apnea is diagnosed when there are repeated episodes of partial or complete blockage of the airway during sleep. This causes the body's oxygen levels to fall and causes sleep to become fragmented. Each time we fall asleep, the muscles in the back of the throat relax. A child with apnea may have muscles that relax too much, and when this is combined with enlarged tonsils or adenoids, the airway may become blocked when the child is asleep.

Your child *may* have sleep apnea if he or she:

- snores most nights

- has breathing pauses or appears to hold his or her breath while asleep

- has noisy breathing or makes some snorting, choking, or gasping sounds at night

- has chronic congestion or frequent infections of ears or sinuses

- breathes through his or her mouth and has a dry mouth in the morning

- has very restless sleep (although *many* children are very restless at night)

- gets hot or sweaty at night (although *many* children get overheated at night)

- tries to sleep in an unusual position; for example, with his or her head elevated or propped up against the head of the bed

- has a large tongue, large tonsils, or large adenoids

- is overweight

- wets the bed past the age of six or seven

- sleepwalks or has frequent night terrors

- has a headache in the morning

- has a medical condition such as Down syndrome or cerebral palsy

- has behavioral problems during the day

- is hard to wake in the morning or is sleepy in the daytime

- is hyperactive or has difficulty paying attention

About 3 to 12 percent of children snore, and about 1 to 10 percent of children have sleep apnea. However, the majority of children with sleep apnea have only mild symptoms and many outgrow this problem without any treatment.

Remember, too, that the last two symptoms in the list above (being sleepy in the daytime or being hyperactive with difficulty focusing) can also be associated with the sleep deprivation that comes from not knowing how to fall asleep quickly and easily at bedtime and not knowing how to return easily to sleep at night. Sometimes these issues can be resolved by teaching your child how to get plenty of sleep by using the five-step plan in this book.

However, if you have concerns about your child's breathing at night, be sure to talk these concerns over with your pediatrician before you begin sleep coaching so that you can feel confident about proceeding. Sleep apnea not only causes frequent awakenings at night, but it can also lead to slower growth and development, attention-related problems, hyperactivity, learning issues, and other medical problems.

Your pediatrician can order a sleep study for your child to confirm or rule out sleep apnea. You can read more about how to prepare your child for a sleep study in Appendix A. If sleep apnea is confirmed, you may want your child to see an ENT (ear, nose, and throat) specialist who can evaluate whether surgery to remove your child's tonsils and adenoids might be helpful.

Sleep apnea, if undiagnosed, can worsen sleep and negatively affect school performance. Sometimes a teacher may think that a child has ADHD when the child actually has sleep apnea or another sleep disorder! So before starting your child on any medications for ADHD, be sure to rule out sleep apnea. ADHD medication can have negative effects on sleep and appetite and can cause anxiety, behavioral problems and dependence so it's important to make sure sleep apnea isn't the root of the problem.

Restless Legs Syndrome (RLS) is a condition that causes uncomfortable sensations in the legs. Your child might report, for example, that he needs to move his legs a lot as he is falling asleep. He might seem restless or fidgety and might have a hard time falling asleep. He might even say something like "it feels like bugs or ants are crawling inside my legs" or "my legs feel tingly." This sensation may cause your child to want to stretch or move his legs a lot in bed, or he may even want to get up and walk around because movement often brings some relief. A child with restless legs syndrome will often have a close relative with this condition, too. RLS may be present more frequently in children with a diagnosis of ADHD as well.

If you think your child may have restless legs syndrome, talk to your pediatrician. A test to check your child's ferritin (iron) levels will often be the next step. If your child's ferritin is low, your pediatrician is likely to want you to give your child iron supplementation or perhaps another type of medication. You will also want to make sure your child is getting enough sleep and avoiding caffeine.

Head banging and **body rocking** are ways that some children comfort themselves while falling asleep. These may sound unusual but these movements are seen in many healthy infants and very young children so this is usually not considered a medical sleep disorder. Most children over the age of three have outgrown these behaviors but 5 percent or so of five-year-old children, for example, still use these types of movements to comfort themselves at night. If these behaviors do not end soon after age five, the child may have some type of developmental delay, autism, or a neurological problem. You should always talk with your child's pediatrician, of course, if you have concerns.

You probably won't need to worry about protecting your child during these behaviors since most children are not likely to harm themselves. You may want to consider moving the bed away from the wall to reduce any noise associated with these behaviors or installing a padded headboard. You may also want to make sure that any hardware on the bed stays tightly connected since these rhythmic behaviors can sometimes cause hardware to loosen. You can also let your child sleep on a low bed on a carpeted floor. Children who have some type of developmental delay, autism, or neurological issue may benefit from wearing a soft foam helmet at nighttime or may need to sleep in a bed with a special kind of strong net around it.

Three-year-old Max sat up in bed and rocked at night for long periods to soothe himself to sleep. His mother thought that it would be best for him if she laid him back down each time this happened. She was sure that he would rock the rest of the night if she did not do this. Since this was happening four or more times a night, his mother was getting exhausted.

Max had already had a neurological workup and an overnight sleep study and neither revealed any problem. Since body rocking is usually not harmful to a child, Max's mother began letting him sleep with lots of pillows around him on a twin mattress on the carpeted floor of his bedroom. His mother stopped going in at night to lay him back down. His mother still watched him on a video monitor from her own room for a few more weeks and noticed that he always laid back down after a period of time. He began waking less often and did not hurt himself in any way with this new arrangement. His mother soon felt much better about his body rocking and about his ability to get restful sleep, and she slept better herself without needing to get up so often at night.

Bruxism is another name for teeth grinding. One-third to one-half of young children grind their teeth at night and most are under the age of 5. Usually this issue is mild, and almost all children outgrow this, but you can do your part by making sure your child drinks plenty of water and is not vitamin deficient (especially in calcium or vitamin B). Also, make sure that your child does not consume much caffeine (in sodas, for example). Sometimes children who snore or have sleep apnea grind their teeth, too. Others might have teeth that do not fit together well or may be teething. Again, most children outgrow bruxism, and unless your child's pediatrician or dentist is concerned about this behavior you do not need to worry too much about this issue.

10

Could My Anxious Child Become a Better Sleeper?

Six-year-old Zora became anxious and clingy as bedtime neared. She often stalled when it was time to go upstairs for her bath, and she dawdled through toothbrushing time. She asked for many more books after reading time was supposed to be over and would go to sleep only while holding her mother's hand. Even if her mother sat right next to the bed and held her hand, Zora might report that her animal wall decals were "looking at her" or that she heard a sound outside. She might even report a tummy ache or a "weird feeling in her legs," even though she had seemed fine just before bedtime. Over time, Zora's mother realized that Zora did not know how to fall asleep independently, and this was making Zora feel very fearful near bedtime.

It's important for you to know that children often behave in ways similar to Zora if they do not know how to fall asleep on their own. Children almost *have to* report various kinds of concerns because they really need their parents to stay close by until they fall asleep. If you think about it, you may have unintentionally trained your child to develop and use anxious behaviors because that's the only way your child can keep you from leaving, especially if he or she does not feel confident about his or her ability to fall asleep independently.

As you work your way through the five-step plan in this book, you can feel confident that you are providing all of the things your child needs at bedtime to feel cozy and comfortable. This five-step plan is designed to reduce anxiety in your child in several ways. It includes a snack to make sure your child isn't hungry, recommends some time spent reading and cuddling, provides a security object and a toy or book for your child to use to relax with until he or she is drowsy enough to fall asleep, and gives your child two bedtime tickets for anything that might have been forgotten. Finally, it gives your child your presence nearby at first while she is mastering the skill of falling asleep independently at bedtime.

Is Your Child's Anxiety at Bedtime Real?

If you are not sure if your child's anxiety around bedtime is real, or whether it is something she reports to avoid falling asleep independently, ask yourself several questions.

- Does your child report many more fears at bedtime than in the daytime?

- Does your child express fear to only one parent and not to the other? In other words, is your child reporting anxiety only when one parent and not the other is putting her to bed?

- Does your child fall asleep quickly and without much fear if someone lies down with her?

If any of these are the case, your child may be reporting anxiety simply because she does not yet know how to fall asleep independently. Your child may be reporting this fear to keep you nearby, since she hasn't yet mastered this skill.

Does Your Child Become Anxious When the Bedtime Routine Ends?

If your child tends to be anxious, you may need to use a much more gradual approach when you are helping him or her become a better sleeper, especially while you are teaching your child to self-soothe as detailed in Chapter 6.

Once you are ready to set limits at bedtime, you may worry that this, too, will make your child more anxious. However, please remember that children are usually much more anxious when they don't know how (or when) the bedtime routine will end, and when they don't know how to fall asleep independently. If you want your child to be calm and relaxed instead of clingy and anxious at bedtime, it is imperative to teach your child good sleep skills and set clear limits. Once this happens, your child will be much more confident about his or her ability to fall asleep anywhere and in almost any setting.

Are You Unwittingly Rewarding Your Child's Anxious Behaviors?

Take a good look at your behaviors, too, if you are concerned about anxiety in your child. You might, without meaning to, of course, be rewarding your child's reports of being anxious or frightened by giving him lots more soothing, attention, and time when he reports these feelings. If reporting fear results in your child getting to sleep in your bed or convinces you to lie down in his bed, your child is sure to go on reporting these feelings to you.

Important note: Some parents have never thought of it this way, but a child really has no other choice but to act afraid or to report feeling anxious if he or she has not yet been taught to fall asleep independently. This is the only way a child can make sure a parent will stay to provide the help he or she currently needs.

Many parents find that a child who has been labeled as anxious becomes much more confident at bedtime and during the day, too, once he or she learns good sleep skills. Children are often more capable than parents think they are. Your child will quickly learn good sleep skills if you express your confidence in him or her and are consistent in your use of the five-step plan. During the day it can be easier to ignore fear and worry (for adults, too!), but when it's time for you to leave after the bedtime routine concludes, what should you do if your child becomes anxious? Remember, if your child is lying in bed without much to do, your child may have a much more difficult time dealing with his or her anxious feelings. That is why the five-step plan recommends giving your child a Bedtime Buddy and a Bedtime Basket to use until he or she is drowsy enough to fall asleep.

If your child asks to leave her bed to come to *your* bed when she is afraid, try to avoid this because you are, in a way, teaching your child that *her bed* is an unsafe place to be. You also want the shift from feeling anxious to feeling relaxed to happen in your child's room rather than in yours, so take your child back to her own room and then help her fall back to sleep.

Is Your Child Afraid of Monsters or Other Scary Things at Night?

If your child talks about being afraid of monsters, robbers, kidnappers, or bad guys around bedtime, try not to give too much attention to these fears. And don't ever add any "monster" steps (like checking for monsters under the bed, using "monster spray," and so on) to the routine since there aren't any monsters in your home! Simply say, "You are safe in our home, and we will always take care of you." If your child insists that someone needs to check for monsters, offer to check only one or two spots to avoid any stalling of the routine.

If your child continues to insist on this after you've reassured him or her by checking a couple of spots, try saying, "I've checked but you can check other spots if you like. Just call me back when you are finished. You're always safe here in our home!" Then step away for a few moments. Your child will be more reassured in the long run with this approach and he or she is likely to stop talking about monsters so often since he or she certainly doesn't want you to leave in the middle of the bedtime routine. You can discuss your child's fears during the day, of course. You can help your child explore these and plan ways to deal with them, but bedtime is not the time to focus on these fears.

Fear of the Dark

If your child is afraid of the dark, remember the bedtime routine in this book recommends both a nightlight and a small reading light. The reading light may be left on all night as long as it is not too bright.

Fear of the Bedroom

If your child has a fear of his or her own bedroom, you can make a list of fears in order of the easiest to manage to the hardest and then you can help your child get more comfortable with each step until he or she feels safe and secure in his or her room again.

For example, your child's list might include:

- being in his or her bedroom with a parent and with the lights on,

- being in his or her bedroom with a parent and with the lights off,

- being in his or her bedroom alone with the lights on, and

- being in his or her bedroom alone with a night-light and a reading light on.

One way to help your child work through this fear is to stay on each step until your child feels comfortable. When you get to the step that has him spending time alone in his room with only the nightlight and the reading light on, you can try doing flashlight treasure hunts. With this technique, you would put a small reward in his room and send him in to find this reward while you wait in the doorway. Over time, you can make the reward harder and harder to find.

Is Your Child Worrying in Bed?

For a child who worries in bed, try establishing a "worry time" in the daytime instead. Worry time is a designated time during the day for your child to talk with you about any worries he or she might have. Usually, thirty minutes is set aside. If your child runs out of worries before this time is up, the remaining time is used to play a game, do a craft, or read together. This technique is meant to teach your child there is a time and a place for worry and, more importantly, that the bed should not be used as a "worry place." If a child brings up a worry before or after worry time, he or she can write it down on an index card and put it in a "worry time box" to save it for worry time.

11

Dealing with Nightmares, Night Terrors, Sleepwalking, and Bedwetting

In this chapter, we will talk about some of the most common sleep-related problems: nightmares, night terrors, sleepwalking, and bedwetting, and discuss how to deal with these.

How Should I Deal with My Child's Nightmares or Night Terrors?

A nightmare is a bad dream that causes a child to wake up with feelings of fear. Nightmares are very common in young children. Most will seek out a parent after a nightmare and most will also recall them in the morning. Nightmares usually occur later in the night when there is more dream sleep.

A night terror seems similar to a nightmare, but a child will not have any memory of the night terror in the morning. During a night terror, a child might have his or her eyes open, sit up in bed, leave the bed, scream or shout, or act frightened. A child will often seem confused, and he or she usually cannot be comforted by a parent. After a period of time (usually ten to thirty minutes), the child will calm down and go back to sleep. Night terrors usually occur during the first few hours of sleep.

Both nightmares and night terrors tend to occur more often if a child is sleep deprived. Let's talk a bit more about both of these.

Nightmares

If your child has nightmares or bad dreams *occasionally*, these are not cause for concern. These are part of normal childhood development. If your child reports nightmares or bad dreams almost every night around bedtime, remember that nightmares usually occur during the second half of the night. This is important to remember because if your child is reporting these just after you leave or perhaps just an hour or so later, your child may be reporting them as an "admission ticket" to your bed.

The plan in this book should soon result in more sleep, which should help to significantly decrease nightmares since they are more frequent in sleep-deprived children or those with inconsistent sleep schedules. Nightmares might also occur more frequently if your child goes to bed with a full stomach, so be sure dinner is eaten well before bedtime and that the bedtime snack is light.

You can teach your child some skills to deal with nightmares, too, by teaching your child to be in charge of his or her dreams. For example, you can help your child re-script the content of the bad dream during the day and read this new version out loud one-half hour before bed. You can end the new script with a powerful statement like, "Even when monsters come after me in my dream, I have so many superpowers!"

If you continue to be concerned about your child's nightmares after your child is obtaining adequate sleep, please discuss this further with your child's pediatrician.

Night Terrors

Remember, a night terror, unlike a nightmare, is something *your child will not remember in the morning*, so your main job is to keep your child safe during these events and not to wake him or her.

Night terrors can be more frequent if your child is sleep deprived, has an inconsistent sleep schedule or a new daytime schedule, has sleep apnea, is sick, has a full bladder, or is sleeping in a new setting. Sometimes noises or lights (or even stress from a new situation) can trigger these. Most children outgrow night terrors by age four or so. Night terrors usually happen during the first few hours of sleep.

If your child has night terrors frequently (many nights a week), and if these occur around the same time each night, you might want to try **scheduled awakenings**. To try this technique, track the time that your child has a night terror for a couple of weeks and, if it does often occur at the same time, try going to your child about fifteen minutes prior to the usual episode. Gently awaken your child by speaking his or her name in a soft voice until your child flutters his or her eyelids or changes position, and then gently encourage him or her to drop right back off to sleep. Scheduled awakenings often result in a decrease in night terrors if used consistently for two to four weeks. If they do not, remember that your main job during a night terror is simply to keep your child safe.

What If My Child Sleepwalks?

Eight-year-old Adam's parents brought him in for a sleep evaluation because he had actually walked right out of his home in the middle of the night and had been found by a neighbor three doors down. His family was terrified that he would do it again and wanted to know how to keep him safe. They wanted to learn how to keep him from sleepwalking at all, if they could, and they also wanted to do everything they could to provide a safe sleep environment for Adam if he did sleepwalk again.

Sleepwalking is a normal part of childhood, and up to 40 percent of children sleepwalk at some point. Most of the time, this behavior disappears by puberty. One study surveyed parents of eighteen hundred children in Australia, and these parents noted that 10 percent of their children (ages five to ten years old) had sleepwalked in the previous week. As common as this issue is, however, sleepwalking can be dangerous. There are several things you can do to keep sleepwalking to a minimum and to provide a safe sleep environment for your child.

How Can I Keep Sleepwalking to a Minimum?

Make sure your child is getting enough sleep (and be sure you have finished the job of helping your child learn to fall asleep independently). Sleepwalking is *much* more common in sleep-deprived children and in those with inconsistent sleep schedules. It's also more common in children who require a lot of time to fall asleep at bedtime. Finally, it's more often seen in children whose parents leave the child's room *after* the child has fallen asleep. All children wake up several times during the night, usually at the end of a sleep cycle. If there is something missing, such as the presence of a parent who was there at bedtime, this can trigger a sleepwalking episode.

How Can I Keep My
Sleepwalking Child Safe?

If your child sleepwalks, your most important job as a parent is to provide a safe environment. You must have a way to be immediately aware that your child is on the move at night. You can install a motion sensor with an alarm in your child's bedroom doorway. This will sound an alarm if your child leaves the bedroom.

A bed alarm can be an even better choice. This alarm consists of a pad that is placed under the fitted sheet of your child's bed and is connected to an alarm by a cord that is usually a few feet long. This cord and alarm can be placed under your child's bed, hung on the headboard, or mounted on the wall. When your child leaves the bed, the alarm will sound to alert you. You can then come to your child's room, silence the alarm, help your child back to bed, and reset the alarm each time this behavior occurs. You can also put a baby monitor in the master bedroom to make sure you hear the bed alarm at night because children are very deep sleepers and your child is not likely to hear it.

This type of alarm is recommended because it can go wherever your child goes. Your child is especially at risk of sleepwalking while on a sleepover, in a hotel, at summer camp, at a relative's home, or anytime he or she sleeps away from home in a new environment. This bed alarm can be used in any of these environments. You will need to be sure that any adults who will be responsible for your child know exactly how to use this alarm.

Other home safety measures are recommended as well. You will want to install gates at the top of any stairways; add nightlights in the hallways; alarm and secure all exit doors and windows; and perhaps install high deadbolts on all exit doors as well. You will also want to keep floors and hallways clutter-free.

When you intercept your sleepwalking child, just guide him or her back to bed. Don't try to wake your child since this can be more distressing. It's not really necessary to talk with your child about the sleepwalking episode the next day since he or she will be unaware of it. Talking about these episodes too much may make your child feel embarrassed or maybe even frightened about going to bed.

What Else Can I Do About Sleepwalking?

Try scheduled awakenings. Track the time your child sleepwalks for a couple of weeks and, if he or she often sleepwalks at the same time, try going to your child about fifteen minutes prior to the usual episode. Gently awaken your child by speaking his or her name in a soft voice until your child flutters his or her eyelids or changes position, and then gently encourage him or her to drop right back off to sleep.

Evaluate your child's room at the time that he or she often sleepwalks. Is there a noise that occurs right around that time? Perhaps there is a neighbor that arrives home from a late shift and slams a car door, for example. Does a pet jump onto or off of your child's bed? Is the sleepwalking episode tied to a time when your child might need to urinate? Be sure you've addressed all of these causes, and feel free to add a fan or white noise machine to your child's room to mask ambient noises in the home or neighborhood.

Treat bedwetting if your child is still wetting the bed after age seven. Some children sleepwalk when their bladder is too full at night.

What If My Child Wets the Bed?

Ten-year-old Ryan was still wetting the bed each night. He really wanted to learn how to stop bedwetting because he wanted to go on sleepovers or away to summer camp without needing a pull-up. Ryan was feeling embarrassed about this problem, and he avoided sleeping away from home.

Ryan's pediatrician had suggested the use of a medication to help with this problem, but this did not work for him. His mother tried restricting how much liquid he drank after 7 p.m., but this did not help either. Finally, she tried waking him to urinate at night when she went to bed (and sometimes again in the middle of the night), but even this did not help Ryan to be reliably dry all the time.

Ryan and his mother decided to try something that almost always works well: a moisture-sensing bedwetting alarm. Ryan and his mom were excited to try it because his pediatrician told him that using this type of alarm is often the best and fastest way to treat this issue.

The pediatrician also told them that most kids who wet the bed past the age of seven are very deep sleepers. These deep sleepers almost never wake up when the alarm goes off, so Ryan's mom knew responding to the alarm was entirely her job and that the more quickly she responded, the more successful Ryan would be.

When the alarm arrived in the mail, Ryan and his mom opened the box and unwrapped the alarm. It was the size and shape of a small tape measure and had a clip that allowed it to be attached to Ryan's underwear. He then put on a pull-up over his underwear so that cleanup after any accidents would be quick and simple.

When Ryan first started using the alarm, his mother slept near him in a spare bed so that she would be sure to hear the alarm. Later when he was dry more often, she put a monitor in her room so she could sleep in her own bed but still listen for the alarm. When the alarm sounded at night, she went to Ryan as quickly as she could, called his name, and asked him to stand up and walk to the bathroom. She repeated this each and every night, teaching him to finish urinating in the toilet if any urine was still left in his bladder and then to change into dry underwear, reattach the alarm, and put on a new pull-up.

After using the alarm every night for about six weeks, Ryan was dry at night. Treating bedwetting with a moisture-sensing alarm usually takes six to eight weeks of very consistent use. After this length of time, children usually either begin to wake up when they need to go to the bathroom or stay dry until morning.

Ryan and his mother also did some other things to help him to maintain his gains. He made sure to go to the bathroom at regular times during the day, and when he did, he would practice starting and stopping the stream of urine. Once he had been dry for two full weeks, he tried using the "overlearning" technique to make sure he would stay dry; he drank eight ounces of water before bed and continued to use the alarm each night until he was dry at night for two more weeks.

Ryan was soon dry all night every night and was so proud and happy about achieving this milestone. His mom signed him up for summer camp with a friend, and Ryan knew he'd be just fine.

Bedwetting is not usually treated with a behavioral plan until after the ages of six or seven since about 10 percent of seven-year-old children are still not reliably dry at night. The rate of bedwetting is usually higher for boys than for girls. It is important to know that this problem is *never* one of laziness or "not trying hard enough." These children sleep so deeply that they do not wake up when they have a full bladder.

Bedwetting in older children can lead to anxiety or a loss of self-esteem; it can also result in children who avoid sleepovers, sleepaway camp, or overnight class trips. However, bedwetting is a very treatable issue.

Moisture-sensing alarms are often the best way to treat bedwetting. These devices are attached to a child's underwear and detect the first drop of wetness and sound an alarm. These alarms are available online or from any large medical supply store. Be sure the alarm has the proper batteries, and have your child practice setting off the alarm by touching a slightly wet paper towel to the alarm sensor to make sure the alarm will go off. (There is no shock or pain associated with the alarm; it simply makes a sound when it gets wet.)

Help your child practice attaching the alarm to the waistband of his or her underwear. Your child can wear cotton underwear with pull-ups over the underwear. Be sure your child practices walking to the bathroom after the alarm sounds (again, by setting off the alarm with a slightly wet cloth).

Get the bedroom ready.

- Be sure there is a light near the bed so that you will be able to help your child move safely from the bed to the bathroom at night when the alarm sounds.

- A washable (or disposable) absorbent pad with a waterproof layer can be placed under your child so that the sheets do not need to be changed. When you are shopping for this pad, you may want to search for a "saddle-style" pad because this type of pad is so easy to put on and take off the bed, holds up to six cups of liquid, and stays in place reliably.

- A pair or two of clean underwear should be placed near the bed.

- A hamper near the bed for wet underwear and for the washable type of absorbent pad is also useful.

- A trashcan can be placed nearby if you are using a disposable absorbent pad.

Now you are ready to use the alarm at night. During the night when the child starts to urinate in bed, the alarm will sound. You must be near enough to hear the alarm right away when it sounds (either by sleeping nearby or by using a monitor in your room), and then you must come quickly to the child's bedside.

Ask your child in a quiet, calm voice to stand up and walk to the bathroom. Repeat this request over and over while helping your child to walk to the bathroom and finish urinating in the toilet if any urine was still left in the bladder. Then your child can put on dry cotton underwear, reattach the alarm, put on a pull-up over the underwear and put a new absorbent pad on the bed.

This cycle is repeated each night for several weeks or until your child is reliably dry every night for two weeks. **It is important to note here that it is the responsibility of the *parent* to come to the child each and every time the alarm sounds.** Caregivers can trade off nights to avoid sleep deprivation, of course.

You can encourage your child to take some ownership in this process but only for the parts that do not require listening for the alarm. (Your child is sleeping too deeply to hear the alarm in most cases.) So for example, you can encourage your child to participate by helping to turn off the alarm, putting on dry underwear and a pull-up, reattaching the alarm, replacing the waterproof pad, and putting the wet pad and underwear into the laundry hamper. Never present any of these steps as punishments! Instead, use rewards for each step and mark your child's progress on a calendar.

Once your child is reliably dry for two weeks, "overlearning" can be used to help your child maintain success since about 40 percent of children may relapse and wet the bed again. After two weeks of dry nights in a row, ask your child to drink 8 ounces of water at bedtime, go to the bathroom one last time, and then be tucked into bed. Your child will continue using the alarm until he or she has again achieved fourteen more dry nights in a row, even after drinking water at bedtime. This overlearning practice reduces relapse by up to 30 percent!

12

Could My Child on the Autism Spectrum Become a Better Sleeper?

The Autism and Developmental Disabilities Monitoring Network (ADDM) at the Centers for Disease Control estimates that 1 to 2 percent of children have autism spectrum disorder. Furthermore (and this will not come as a surprise to most parents with a child on the spectrum), the National Institute of Health (NIH) estimates that between 44 and 86 percent of children with autism have a sleep-related problem. Other children may not have an actual diagnosis of autism but may have some behavioral problems that lead to poor sleep.

Abe's story illustrates some of the key ways parents can use the five-step plan in this book to improve the sleep of children with these types of sleep problems.

Five-year-old Abe was on the autism spectrum and lived with his mother, father, and seven-year-old sister. He had trouble falling asleep at bedtime and trouble staying asleep, too, often waking several times throughout the night. Sometimes he woke as early as 4 a.m. and never went back to sleep.

His parents tried putting him to bed each night around 7 p.m. Once they tucked him in, he made lots of callbacks and curtain calls. His curtain calls often involved requests for food or trips to his sister's room to bang on her door and ask if she was still awake.

His mother and father often brought him more snacks when he requested them, and they also made many trips back to his bedroom to tuck him in again. They usually gave in to his many requests after the bedtime routine was over with the hope that he would finally fall asleep if they gave him everything he asked for. When they did try to set limits and keep him in his bed, he might throw toys or books at them. Sometimes he knocked over lamps in his room or even tried to bite or hit his parents. His parents tried using a gate to keep him in his room, but he repeatedly kicked or knocked the gate down.

Once Abe had been persuaded to stay in his room and had quieted down, his parents heard him playing by himself in his room for hours. He got out many of his toys, and sometimes he made so much noise that he woke his sister again.

Abe often did not fall asleep until after 11 p.m., and he was often still awake well after midnight. Once he finally fell asleep, he awoke several times a night and came to his parent's room. They redirected him back to his room each time, but this pattern resulted in lots of lost sleep for both Abe and his parents. He also woke up in the morning between 4 and 5 a.m. no matter when he fell asleep.

Abe's parents were exhausted, to say the least, and were ready to use the five-step plan to help Abe become a better sleeper.

As part of Step 1—preparing your child's bedroom for great sleep—his parents made his room into a large, safe space, almost like a spacious crib. They took off the regular door to his room and, as a sturdy alternative to a gate, replaced it with a half-height door. They also installed a motion sensor that would chime anytime this door was opened.

Abe already had a fun and colorful fish-shaped reading light on his bedside table that he loved, and his parents added a wicker basket to his bedside table to hold a few books and quiet toys. They purchased several toy bins so that they could put the majority of his toys away each night by moving these bins into his closet at bedtime. They added a childproof knob to his closet door so that he could not open the closet once the toys were put away.

They made sure he could not climb on or tip over any of his furniture. They removed floor lamps, cords, and anything else of concern in his room, too. They secured his windows so that they could be opened only a few inches. They had never allowed electronics in his room in the first place, so they had none of these to remove.

They helped him choose a security object to snuggle with each night, and Abe chose his stuffed animal puppy, Fido. His parents began including Fido in every step of the 5B Bedtime Routine.

As part of Step 2—using the 5B Bedtime Routine every night—they made sure Abe had a substantial bedtime snack as the first step in his routine. Once they began making sure Abe had both a good dinner and this healthy bedtime snack each night, his parents did not grant any other requests for food until breakfast time the next morning. They no longer allowed him to take food to his room so that his room was no longer associated with eating.

After his snack, bath, toothbrushing, and final bathroom trip, they chose three or four toys and a couple of books for his bedtime basket and reminded him that he could read and play with these in bed at night by the light of his beloved fish lamp until he was drowsy enough to fall asleep. They put the rest of his toys into bins and put the bins in the closet with the childproof knob.

Once he was tucked into bed with Fido and his basket with a limited set of books and toys, his mother or father read with him for a few minutes until the timer chimed, as long as he did not get out of bed or try to hurt them. Once the timer chimed, the parent on duty for the evening gave Abe a final hug and kiss and sat in a chair in his doorway, allowing Abe to self-comfort with Fido and his Bedtime Basket. A parent stayed in the doorway reading or working without talking until Abe was deeply asleep. If Abe got out of bed, his mother or father tucked him in again only twice. If he came out of bed a third time, his mother or father moved the chair into the hallway, closed the half-height door, and sat in the hallway until he fell asleep. If he fell asleep on his beanbag chair or on his rug instead of in his bed, his mother or father moved him back to his bed much later.

His parents also moved the chair to the hallway and shut the half-height door if he talked to them repeatedly or if he tried to hit or bite them. A parent always stayed nearby until he was deeply asleep during the first few weeks of using the new plan.

If Abe awakened again at night, he would find his half-height door closed and, if he opened the door and came out of his room, the motion sensor would chime. This chime alerted his parents and often gave one of his parents enough time to come to his room and direct him back to his own bed before he made it all the way to the master bedroom.

Abe's parents knew that children on the spectrum often sleep less than other children the same age, so they began tracking how many hours he slept each night once he was used to the new plan and was falling asleep more quickly and easily. They discovered he never slept more than a total of eight hours. Armed with this information, they moved his bedtime snack to 9:30 p.m. and finished up his routine by 10 p.m. each night (instead of the 7 p.m. time they had been using). Abe began sleeping consistently from 10 p.m. to 6 a.m. each night with this new bedtime. This sleep schedule matched theirs, and it worked well for both Abe and his parents since Abe did not wake up so often and so early.

Once firmer limits were being set for Abe at bedtime, and he had learned to play quietly in bed until he was drowsy enough to fall asleep, his parents were able to leave his room each night when the routine was over and enjoy movies together in the living room as a couple. Abe was sleeping deeply and well and so were his parents and his sister.

Bedtime Stories:
How Some Real Kids
Learned to Be Great Sleepers

If you have a child with sleep problems, you already know you are far from alone! So many parents struggle with these problems. I hope the five-step plan in this book will make you a successful sleep coach for your child. Sometimes it can be helpful to see how other parents reached this goal. This epilogue is included in the book so you can read some stories about exactly how parents and caregivers in my practice have used the five-step plan for their children. I hope you find stories here that address some of the issues your child is having. If so, I hope the stories provide you with even more specific ideas about how you can be a successful sleep coach for your own child.

Leo, Who Had a Two-Hour Bedtime Routine

Leo, a six-year-old who had a hard time falling asleep every night, usually began stalling just before bedtime. "Mom, I'm not sleepy at all yet!" he would say. Or "Can I stay up late tonight with you and Dad?" Even after his parents finally got him into bed, Leo wanted even more help from his parents in order to fall asleep.

On a typical night, Leo might ask, "Dad, would you read me one more story?" or "Mom, I just can't sleep. Will you rub my back for a while?" After his parents finally slipped out of his room, hoping to relax in the living room and watch a movie together, Leo was sure to come out of his bedroom again to tell them one more thing, to get one more kiss, to give them one more hug, or to ask for one more drink of water (even though he had to pass right by a faucet to find his parents!).

Once his parents had granted all of these requests and thought Leo was finally asleep, he often came out of his room again to report more problems: "My bed feels hot!" or "I need to go to the bathroom again! Can you come with me?"

On rare nights, Leo might finally doze off on his own, but most of the time he just could not fall asleep independently. His bedtime routine lasted more than two hours and included many callbacks and curtain calls after lights out. His parents granted all these requests because they hoped if Leo finally had everything he needed, he would get down to the business of falling asleep. However, nothing seemed to reliably send him off to dreamland, so each night around ten o'clock, after a long struggle, his parents finally gave up, and one of them agreed to lie in his bed with him and rub his back to relax him. Once this happened, Leo fell asleep almost instantly.

By granting all of Leo's extra requests after the bedtime routine ended, Leo's parents had, without meaning to, been rewarding him for staying up later. The longer it took him to fall asleep, the more attention he received from his parents! Without intending to, they had been teaching him to fall asleep only when they were present because he almost never fell asleep until they finally gave up and came to his room to stay.

Besides resulting in a bedtime routine that lasted for hours and exhausted everyone, this routine also caused several other problems. Each time Leo woke up during the night, he called out for a parent to come back to his room and lie down with him again in order to fall back to sleep. Leo was also often tardy for school because he fell asleep so late that his parents worried about waking him up too early in the morning. Leo also missed out on the sleepovers his other friends enjoyed because he did not feel confident about his ability to fall asleep independently away from home. Finally, Leo's parents felt frustrated that they never had time to themselves to relax and recharge.

Ready to make changes to help Leo become a great sleeper, his parents decided to do some sleep coaching with Leo. They prepared his room for great sleep by putting a reading lamp and a nightlight in his bedroom and helping him choose his favorite stuffed animal, Zoe the Zebra, as his Bedtime Buddy. They also put a book into his Bedtime Basket along with another quiet toy, his favorite tiny fire engine.

They used the 5B Bedtime Routine each night, and they let him know that, when reading time was over, they would lie in his bed at night until he fell asleep. However, they also let him know that they would be silent during this time while he played with Zoe, or looked at the book, or played with his tiny fire engine. They told him they would not rub his back and that over time they would be moving farther away from him (from the bed to a chair and so on).

On the first night of the new routine, while Leo's mother put Leo's baby brother to sleep, Leo's father followed the bedtime routine, being sure to include Zoe the Zebra every step of the way. Leo's dad gave him a bedtime snack in the kitchen and supervised a bath, toothbrushing, and a final bathroom trip. Then he, Leo, and Zoe curled up to read in Leo's bed and set a timer to mark the end of reading time. He then tucked Leo into bed next to Zoe and gave Leo his two Bedtime Tickets along with his Bedtime Basket. Leo's father reminded Leo that he could read his book or play with his fire engine quietly until he felt ready to fall asleep.

After granting one more request when Leo decided to redeem a Bedtime Ticket for a different book, his father laid down in Leo's bed with a body pillow between them and discouraged any further interactions by reading his own book. Leo played quietly with his small fire engine for only about five minutes and then dropped off to sleep.

Each night after Leo fell deeply asleep, his father left his room and joined Leo's mother in the living room where they enjoyed some relaxing time together. Each morning, Leo usually had one Bedtime Ticket left to trade for a small reward. His favorite reward was doing a special craft project with his mom after school.

After one week of this new routine, Leo's father moved out of Leo's bed at the end of reading time and sat in a chair right next to Leo's bed. Leo grumbled a bit about this at first, but his father knew Leo was ready for the next step and told Leo how proud he was of the progress he had already made. Leo's father continued to read his own book while Leo played quietly on his own in bed until he felt drowsy enough to fall asleep. After two weeks, Leo's father moved the chair to the doorway of Leo's room and, one week later, Leo's father was able to leave Leo's room immediately after reading time was over.

Leo became a pro at falling asleep on his own. Once he learned that his parents gave him very little attention after he used his Bedtime Tickets, there was nothing left to do but play for a few minutes and then fall asleep. Leo tried to make the most of a Bedtime Ticket one night by asking his parents if he could use one to order a take-out pizza, but his parents reminded him that Bedtime Tickets were only good for a quick request!

Leo soon fell asleep much earlier in the evening and felt confident about his ability to relax himself to sleep at bedtime. He stayed in his room without coming to find his parents if he woke up at night, too, because he had learned to fall asleep on his own so easily at bedtime. He soon became able to get up on time for school as well. Leo's parents felt great about their sleep coaching skills. Leo was very proud of his accomplishments, too, because he could finally go on birthday party sleepovers. He even felt confident enough to begin making plans with friends to go to a sleep-away camp the next summer.

Amanda, Who Slept with a Menagerie of Stuffed Animals

Amanda was five years old and loved her cute and colorful menagerie of stuffed animals. At bedtime, she would not get into bed unless at least a dozen of these were set up at the foot of her bed. If any of her favorites were missing, they had to be found. If any of them fell over, they had to be set up again before she would lie down.

Once her stuffed animals were settled, Amanda's mother would leave Amanda's room to put the baby to sleep, and Amanda's father would rub her back and read to her until she fell asleep.

Her father stopped reading when he thought Amanda was asleep, but Amanda often sat right up again to ask him to keep reading. Reading her to sleep often took well over an hour. During the middle of the night, each time Amanda awoke, she would call her father back to set her stuffed animals up again or to read again. This happened many times a night, and both Amanda and her father were becoming very sleep-deprived.

When Amanda's father was ready to improve her sleep and her bedtime routine, he asked Amanda to choose only two of these animals to be part of her bedtime routine that night. Only these two animals participated in the steps in the 5B Bedtime Routine and were tucked in with her instead of being set up at the foot of the bed.

Next, Amanda's father continued to read to her each night but only until the timer chimed. Amanda then looked at books independently until she was able to fall asleep on her own. Amanda was soon going to sleep much more quickly and with much less stress. She also stopped waking up so often at night, and when she did wake up, her father came to her room and reminded her to cuddle her animals until she was able to fall back to sleep.

Mira, Who Stayed Up Until the Hospital Night Shift Started

Mira's mother was an emergency room physician who worked a night shift, leaving for work around 10:15 p.m. each night. Even though Mira, a four-year-old, had a great bedtime routine that wrapped up around 8 p.m., Mira would call her mother back for all kinds of reasons so that she'd be able to stay awake until her mother left for work.

Mira's mother knew she needed to work out a new bedtime routine to help Mira fall asleep earlier. Since Mira loved puzzles, she and her mom began spending time putting puzzles together after dinner, and then they moved through the steps in her bedtime routine. They concluded the routine by reading together in Mira's bed until 8:30 p.m. Then Mira's mother let Mira know that she would be home in time to have breakfast with Mira in the morning and that only Mira's dad would be responding to any other requests after 8:30 p.m. This encouraged Mira to fall asleep at the appropriate bedtime and to get enough sleep each night. Every morning when Mira woke up, she'd find her mom in the kitchen making a scrumptious breakfast for them to eat together. Sometimes, since she'd fallen asleep at her ideal bedtime, they even had time to play and do puzzles together again for a while before Mira left for school.

Tasha, Whose Mother
Had "Tried Everything"

Four-year-old Tasha's mom often worried about how little sleep Tasha was getting, even though she had tried everything to help Tasha become a great sleeper. She made sure that Tasha turned off electronics one hour before bed. She worked hard to make Tasha's bedroom a perfect sleep environment. She put an aromatherapy diffuser in her room to waft the scent of lavender flowers near her bed. She bought Tasha a specially shaped pillow and a weighted blanket. She added a light that made the constellations revolve on Tasha's ceiling.

When this didn't seem to help, she added a fan and a sound machine that played ocean waves. If the sound of the ocean did not seem to help, Tasha's mother would try lullabies or meditation tapes made for children. She replaced the white lightbulbs in Tasha's room with pink ones that cast a warm glow and contained none of the blue light that might make Tasha more wakeful at night.

When Tasha still could not fall asleep easily, her mother began giving Tasha warm chocolate milk in bed followed by a back massage. Despite all of this, Tasha was still not sleeping well.

Tasha's mother had, without meaning to, created a bedtime routine that was ever-changing and was actually more entertaining than calming. Tasha never knew what to expect at bedtime because her mother kept adding more interesting items to her bedroom and more steps to her bedtime routine. This inconsistency actually made it harder for Tasha to fall asleep. And the longer it took Tasha to fall asleep, the more wonderful things she received (back rubs, soft music, warm cocoa, and so on).

Tasha's bedtime routine not only wasn't working well, but it was also taking a loooong time. Hours after the bedtime routine began, Tasha finally fell asleep only when her mother lay down next to her. She left after Tasha fell asleep, but Tasha often woke again just after midnight. She would call for her mother who then returned to her room to repeat many of the same steps she had used at bedtime to get Tasha back to sleep. This routine often had to be repeated once again in the wee hours of the morning.

Meanwhile at preschool (to her mother's bewilderment), Tasha fell asleep each day during naptime with a very simple routine: she retrieved her favorite stuffed giraffe out of her backpack, curled up on her cot, and fell fast asleep in a few moments!

When Tasha's mother was ready to improve her sleep, she worked through the five-step plan. First, Tasha's mother prepared Tasha's bedroom for great sleep by removing the aromatherapy diffuser, star projector, music player, fan, and white noise machine. She added a nightlight and a reading light. Tasha chose her giraffe as her Bedtime Buddy and chose a toy and a favorite picture book for her Bedtime Basket. Tasha and her mother also decorated two Bedtime Tickets with some of Tasha's favorite stickers.

Next, Tasha's mom reviewed the 5B Bedtime Routine and realized that she needed to give Tasha her cocoa in the kitchen as part of the Bedtime Bite. She kept a short backrub as part of the routine but made sure that Tasha did not fall asleep during the backrub by putting it right after the final bathroom trip and right before reading time.

When the reading timer chimed to mark the end of reading time (and the end of the 5B Bedtime Routine), Tasha's mother gave her the Bedtime Basket and her Bedtime Tickets and lay down in bed with Tasha as usual, but after reminding Tasha to read or play until she was drowsy enough to fall asleep, Tasha's mother stayed very quiet. She often acted like she was asleep until Tasha drifted off and then she left Tasha's room to relax and read in the living room.

After a few nights, Tasha's mother put a body pillow between herself and Tasha, and, after a few more nights, she moved to a chair near the bed. Tasha's mother was able to move farther and farther away over time until Tasha could fall asleep independently.

When Tasha woke up at night, her mother came back to her room and sat nearby until Tasha fell back to sleep. Once Tasha had lots of practice falling asleep independently at bedtime, her night wakings virtually disappeared.

James, Who Would Not
Sleep in His Own Bed

Five-year-old James never wanted to go to his bedroom at night. His parents had never really developed a bedtime routine for him, so James fell asleep on the living room sofa while they watched their favorite series on TV every night. If they tried to send him up to bed, he told them that he didn't like to be upstairs when they were downstairs and that his room had a "scary window."

So every night right after dinner, he brought his pillow and favorite blanket down to the living room and curled up on the sofa while his parents did the dishes. He fell asleep on the sofa each night while his parents watched their favorite shows. Once he was deeply asleep, his dad carried him up to bed.

After midnight each night, his parents would hear his footsteps on the stairs as he headed to the living room again to turn the TV back on. They were usually able to intercept him before he made it to the living room and would walk him back to bed. More often, however, they would find him asleep on the living room couch in the morning with the TV on.

James did not have a consistent bedtime routine to help him become drowsy and comfortable in his bedroom, so he had learned to fall asleep easily only by being near his parents on the living room sofa with the TV on. A child without a regular bedtime routine who learns to fall asleep in another part of the house and who is moved to his or her bed later will often try to re-create what was happening at bedtime when they wake up at night by going back to the spot where he or she initially fell asleep. They will also often report that there is something scary about their room or protest being alone there.

James's parents knew they had to find a better way to put him to bed at night. They first worked on preparing his bedroom. They made sure he had a nightlight and a reading light beside his bed along with a cup for water. They put a heavy, dark curtain over the "scary window" and they gave him a keychain flashlight so that he could check the window and every corner of his room from his bed if he wanted to. They helped him choose a Bedtime Buddy, and James chose Leon, his stuffed lion. They filled a Bedtime Basket for him with a couple of his favorite toys and books.

He did have a TV in his room because his parents had tried a few months before to help him learn to fall asleep in his own room with the TV on (instead of in the living room). His parents removed the TV from his room altogether, knowing it would be too hard for James to leave it off at night if he could see it when he went to bed or woke up at night.

Finally, they put a motion sensor on his door because he had a longstanding habit of leaving his room at night to go back to the living room, and they wanted to be sure that they knew right away when he was on the move.

Next they designed a great bedtime routine for him using the 5B Bedtime Routine as their guide, and they added a nice foot rub for him just before they read books together. They included his Bedtime Buddy in each step, too, because he had not really bonded to a stuffed animal before.

After the 5B Bedtime Routine was over, the parent on duty for the night sat in a chair near James. James did not need a parent to lie in bed with him, even though he was in his room instead of the living room, because he had not become accustomed to falling asleep while actually touching a parent. While James relaxed in bed with Leon and something from his Bedtime Basket, his mother or father read in the chair nearby until James fell asleep. Over time, they moved this chair closer and closer to the doorway and then moved it into the hall. For a few weeks, they had to stay on the same floor as James, but soon they were able to say goodnight to him and be anywhere in their home.

At first, after falling asleep at bedtime, James did come out of his room often at night. His parents heard the chime of the motion sensor as he left his room, so they were able to intercept him in the hallway and take him back to bed each time. They encouraged him to snuggle with Leon again, and he was soon fast asleep. James was soon sleeping through the night, and he was proud of his ability to fall asleep on his own in his bedroom. His parents were happy that he could fall asleep without any electronics, too, by simply looking at books or playing quietly in bed. They knew that this would also help him to sleep well at a friend's or relative's home.

Grace, Who Woke the Neighbors at Bedtime

Five-year-old Grace had a million ways to stall things at bedtime. She'd ask for one more show, one more snack, one more minute in the bathtub, or one more blanket. Once she was finally in bed, Grace's mother let Grace play games on a tablet computer, hoping that this would make her sleepy. Instead, Grace played and played these games until it was very late. When her mother finally insisted that it was time to put away the tablet and go to sleep, Grace would throw a tantrum. She would cry and yell at the top of her lungs each time her mother tried to take it away. If her mother tried to end the bedtime routine with book reading, Grace would throw the book onto the floor.

Her mother was afraid that the neighbors in their apartment building would be upset by Grace's crying and yelling and would call the apartment manager to complain. So she always gave in to Grace and let her play games on the tablet long after Grace should have been asleep. There were many nights when Grace did not fall asleep until after midnight.

Once Grace was deeply asleep, her mother slipped the tablet out of her hands and took it to her own bedroom.

But Grace often woke up again during the night and came running down the hall to find her mother and the tablet again. She would lie in her mother's bed and play on the tablet again until she fell back to sleep.

Since Grace fell asleep so late each night, her mother felt she had to let Grace sleep in as late as she could the next day. If it was a school day, Grace was often tardy, and if it was a weekend or holiday, Grace might sleep until 10 a.m.

When Grace's mother was ready to improve her sleep, she contacted each nearby neighbor to let them know she would soon be starting a new five-step sleep coaching plan for Grace on the upcoming Friday night around 7:30 p.m. and told them Grace might do some loud protesting for a few nights while she was learning to fall asleep without a tablet computer.

Grace's mother helped Grace prepare her bedroom for great sleep by filling a Bedtime Basket with some fun, non-electronic things to do; they chose colored pencils, drawing pads, and a new coloring book since Grace loved to color and draw. They chose a special stuffed animal for Grace's Bedtime Buddy (a fuzzy little red fox her grandmother had given her for her birthday).

Grace and her mother made a chart for the bedroom wall with the pictures of the steps in her bedtime routine, and the first step each night was putting the tablet computer away in a desk drawer that could be locked.

Grace's mother started the routine at 7:30 p.m. each night. If Grace stalled during any of the steps, her mother would finish the step for her if necessary and would do this as calmly as she could manage. For example, if Grace stalled during the Bedtime Bite, her mother would set a timer to mark the end of snack time and would put the food away when the timer chimed. If Grace insisted on staying in the tub too long, her mother would set a timer for three more minutes of playtime in the bubbles and then lift her out of the bath, even if Grace did some protesting.

Once they were sitting in Grace's bed, her mom set a timer to mark the end of their reading time together, too. She let her know that if Grace threw the book or got out of bed, their reading time together would be over. If Grace was relaxed and calm, they read together until the reading timer chimed. Then Grace's mother gave her the Bedtime Basket to use in bed on her own until she was drowsy enough to fall asleep. Since Grace's mother had not been lying in her bed at bedtime before they started this new routine, she just sat in a chair in the doorway reading her own book silently until Grace fell deeply asleep to make sure Grace didn't leave her room.

Grace protested loudly and often the first week, but her mother continued to move calmly and confidently through the bedtime routine in the same order each night without getting off track. It took Grace a while to fall asleep each night during the first week because the items in the basket were much less stimulating than the tablet. However, soon Grace was falling asleep around 8:30 p.m. each night without any loud fussing, and she began making it to school on time each morning, too. Grace's teachers told her mother that her attention in class and her behaviors during the day were better than they had ever been.

Aisha, Who Needed Her Bedtime Routine to Be Perfect Every Night

Seven-year-old Aisha was happy and curious during the day. She enjoyed going to school and loved her after-school theater group. But at bedtime Aisha had a lot of difficulty falling and staying asleep.

Aisha's bedtime routine had to be done *just so*, and her preferred routine seemed to get longer and more complicated over time. She wanted a cup of warm milk to drink in bed while she and her mother read together. Her mother had to read her favorite books in the same order and in the same way each night. Once book time was over, Aisha wanted her mother to lie down next to her, hold her hand very tightly, and say goodnight very slowly to Aisha's toes, knees, tummy, chin, nose, eyes, and forehead. Aisha wanted her mother to keep saying goodnight to each part, in order, over and over again, until she fell asleep to the sound of her mother's voice.

If Aisha's mother did any of these things "incorrectly," Aisha wanted her mother to start the routine over. For example, if the milk wasn't the right temperature when Aisha got into bed, if her mother read the book in a "different voice" one night, or if she said goodnight to Aisha's toes, knees, and tummy in the wrong order, Aisha insisted that the entire routine be started again from the very beginning. If her mother wouldn't do this, Aisha became tearful and anxious and couldn't fall asleep.

Even after Aisha did fall asleep and her mother tiptoed out of her room, Aisha slept for only two or three hours and when she woke up and found her mother gone, she ran down the hall to her mother's room and stayed there the rest of the night. If her mother tried to take her back to her own bed to get her back to sleep, Aisha would cry loudly and refuse. This situation resulted in lots of lost sleep for both of them.

By now you know that Aisha's "sleep onset associations" unfortunately all involved the presence of her mother. She had learned to need warm milk made just so by her mother, her mother's hand, and the sound of her mother's voice saying goodnight to different parts of her body in order to fall asleep. Aisha needed so many things at bedtime, and all of them had to be done just so. It became harder and harder for Aisha's mother to "do it right" each night. Worst of all, none of these sleep onset associations were available when

Aisha woke up at night, so Aisha could never get back to sleep on her own either.

You also see by now that there were some limit setting issues at play here, too. Aisha didn't know how to fall asleep without her mother nearby, so she insisted on "do-overs" that kept her mother near her for long periods until Aisha was finally drowsy enough to fall asleep. Aisha's mother didn't want her to cry or get upset around bedtime, so she agreed to start the routine over again before Aisha could get "out of control," as her mother put it. Her mother was afraid to set limits because then Aisha would get upset, be awake for hours, and lose the sleep she would need the next day.

When Aisha's mother was ready to improve her sleep, she first added a reading light and a Bedtime Basket with books and puzzles. She changed their bedtime routine, too, by giving Aisha her glass of warm milk in the kitchen only during the Bedtime Bite part of the routine so that her cup of warm milk was no longer associated with her bed at all (and so she didn't have to reheat it to make it juuuust the right temperature!).

Aisha's mother learned why it was so important not to give in to Aisha's protests after the bedtime routine was over and to be firm with setting limits. Not giving in to Aisha's protests actually created the space Aisha needed to learn to how to fall asleep independently with her new routine. For example, her mother still read to her, but a timer was used to mark the end of reading time so that there was no discussion about whether reading time was over. Aisha's mother also let her know that if she complained about *how* her mother read the book, reading time together would be over, and it would then be time for Aisha to read on her own. Finally, her mother continued to say goodnight to parts of Aisha's body, but she asked Aisha to choose only three parts each night. Her mother did not say these goodnights over again if Aisha objected to the order.

Aisha's mother also learned one more way to manage Aisha's behavior if she began demanding that the routine be started over again at any point. Aisha's mother would leave the bed entirely and stand in the doorway. She let Aisha know that she would not start the routine over and that she would wait there in the doorway until Aisha was quieter and calmer again. Then Aisha's mother would come right back to the step in the routine they had been on.

To work on gradually tapering her presence in Aisha's room, her mother stopped holding Aisha's hand and she put a body pillow between herself and Aisha right after the end of their reading time, so Aisha learned how to fall asleep without being able to touch her mother but could still feel some pressure against the side of her body. Aisha read to herself each night until she was drowsy enough to fall asleep, and her mother stayed nearby but remained very quiet while Aisha learned this skill.

After a few nights, her mother moved out of the bed entirely and sat in a chair next to the bed so that Aisha could learn how to fall asleep without her mother being in the bed at all. The body pillow stayed behind, and Aisha liked having this in her bed each night. Every few nights, Aisha's mother moved the chair farther and farther away from the bed until she was sitting in the doorway. Eventually, she was able to leave Aisha's room entirely after the reading timer chimed, and Aisha read herself to sleep each night.

This plan resulted in a much quicker sleep onset for Aisha and far fewer complaints around bedtime. At first, Aisha's mother had to walk Aisha back to her own bed if she came to her mother's room at night and stay a few moments until Aisha was asleep again. Later, Aisha would wake briefly and then go back to sleep on her own without ever leaving the bed because she had mastered this skill at bedtime.

Anna, Who Had Three Different Bedtime Routines

Three-year-old Anna had difficulty falling asleep at night. Her mother had one way of putting her to sleep, her father had a second way, and her live-in grandmother, who put her to sleep when Anna's parents worked late hospital shifts, had a third way.

Her mother let her fall asleep on the living room sofa while the TV was on and moved Anna to the master bedroom later. Her father let her fall asleep in the master bedroom on his chest while he watched TV, and he moved her to her own spot in the master bed once she was deeply asleep. Her grandmother held her in her arms and rocked her to sleep, and then the two of them slept in her grandmother's bed. Anna had her own beautiful room with a canopied twin bed but refused to ever sleep there at all.

During all three of these methods, Anna resisted falling asleep for more than an hour by talking and kicking her legs. She made many extra requests, too, while her parents or grandmother were trying to get her to sleep, and she often tried to wait up for a different person to put her to bed. Since it took so long for her to get to sleep, she was often still awake very late at night, and she slept in every time she could. She never woke up on her own for school, and mornings were a struggle for the whole family. She was also described as hyperactive by her teachers. (Sleep-deprived children are almost always described by others as hyperactive during the daytime rather than sleepy and lethargic.)

Anna's family wanted to develop a new bedtime routine for her with the hope that she could learn to fall asleep quickly and achieve all the sleep she needed. The family made a commitment to use the 5B Bedtime Routine in the same order every night and to make sure each caregiver did the routine in the same way. They also made sure that the bedtime routine always concluded in Anna's room. Her caregivers alternated nights, and the caregiver on duty read two books to her and then moved to a chair near her bed. Anna was given two Bedtime Tickets for two final requests each night and a reward in the morning for any Bedtime Ticket she didn't use. Once her Bedtime Tickets had been used or expired, the caregiver on duty ignored any additional requests while reminding Anna to read or play with items from her Bedtime Basket until she was drowsy enough to go to sleep.

At first, Anna became even more energetic at bedtime during this new routine, but her parents and grandmother made sure she knew two basic rules: she had to stay in her bed, and she had to play quietly until she was drowsy enough to fall asleep. Once she could fall asleep on her own with very little interaction or delay, her parents and grandmother began moving the chair out of her room gradually until they could leave right away after lights out. Anna began falling asleep much earlier and waking up on her own in the morning.

Oliver, Who Was a Midnight Snacker

Ten-year-old Oliver was being raised by his grandparents. He had Attention Deficit Hyperactivity Disorder (ADHD) and took medicine during the day that helped him pay attention in class, but the medication also reduced his appetite for most of the day.

Oliver had a good bedtime routine and his grandparents could leave his room at night at the end of this routine while he read himself to sleep. However, each night around midnight, he woke up and went straight to the kitchen to eat. Oliver needed more food during the day than he was currently eating, but he had gotten into the habit of eating at a time when he actually should have been sleeping.

When a child (or anyone, for that matter) eats at night, he is, in a sense, setting a "stomach alarm clock" to go off at that time. (The stomach has a sort of "clock" just the way the brain does.) Without meaning to, Oliver had trained his stomach to expect food at midnight each night, and his stomach would reliably wake him at that time.

Oliver and his grandparents began making sure that both his dinner and his Bedtime Bite were substantial and nutritious. Oliver and his grandparents made a list of snacks, and they found some that helped him feel full until breakfast time. His two favorite snacks were nut butter on toast or a big bowl of warm oatmeal with maple syrup and almond milk.

Oliver was soon falling asleep around 9 p.m. and sleeping right through the night.

Henry, Whose Dad Sat in the Driveway at Night

Six-year-old Henry's mom had a very difficult time at bedtime because he wanted to stay up until his father got home. His father often got home at 7 p.m. and was able to spend time with him until his 8 p.m. bedtime, but sometimes his father did not arrive home until well after 8 p.m. It took Henry's mom a long time to get Henry to sleep on these nights because, even if she lay in bed with him, he would try to keep himself awake until his father arrived.

In addition, even if Henry did fall asleep around 8 p.m., he would wake after any creak or noise and then ask his mother if his dad was home yet. When Henry's dad did get home, he would pull his car quietly into the driveway and text Henry's mother to ask whether Henry was asleep. If Henry was not yet asleep, Henry's mother would ask Henry's dad to wait in the car until Henry was deeply asleep, but this might not happen until well after 10 p.m.

Henry's parents knew they needed to work out a new routine for him. They taught Henry that if his father was going to get home anytime after 8 p.m., Henry's father would not be coming up to his room that night. Instead, the two of them would have a video call while his dad was still on the train coming home and the two of them would eat breakfast together the next morning. Henry was soon falling asleep at 8 p.m. every night and waking up much more rested in the morning.

Mia, Who Was Afraid of the Dark

Seven-year-old Mia often told her parents that she was afraid of the dark and did not want to sleep in a dimly lit bedroom. She liked to have her bright overhead light, two nightlights, a salt lamp, and a reading light on at night when she was falling asleep. Mia's mother would turn most of these off later when she herself went to bed, but she would soon hear Mia's footsteps on her wooden floor, running to turn them on again when Mia woke up during the night.

Many kids ask to sleep in a well-lit room, but this type of lighting can also become a kind of sleep crutch. Mia had tried sleeping in a spare bed in her grandmother's room on a weekend visit and had tried to go on a sleepover at her friend Olivia's house, but neither Mia's grandmother nor her friend could sleep in such a bright room.

Mia's mom helped her to work through this fear in two ways. First, Mia's mother set up flashlight treasure hunts for her. She put a small reward in her darkened room and let Mia use a flashlight to find it while she waited in the doorway. Every evening she made the reward a bit harder to find until Mia was much more comfortable in her darker room.

Second, Mia's mom gradually eliminated the lights in her room one by one until Mia could sleep with only a nightlight, a flashlight, and a reading lamp. She gave Mia plenty of quiet activities to do by the light of the reading lamp until Mia became drowsy enough to fall asleep. Mia soon became much more comfortable with her more appropriate bedtime lighting and was soon able to sleep better in her own more dimly lit room and at her friend's and her grandmother's homes, too.

Sofia, Whose Dad Slept in a Purple-Canopied Twin Bed

Six-year-old Sofia was often anxious at bedtime. Her mom often lay down with her in her beautiful, purple-canopied twin bed and stayed until Sofia was asleep. Each night around 2 a.m., Sofia would appear in her parents' room and report a nightmare. Her mother would pull her into the middle of the master bed, but Sofia was a very restless sleeper, and her dad began losing sleep because of this pattern. Eventually, he began leaving the bed each night when Sofia came in. He would walk sleepily down the hall to Sofia's bed. He was uncomfortable there and had to curl up on his side with his knees pulled up in order to fit in her small bed, but at least he knew he wouldn't be awakened by her restless movements.

After a few weeks of this, Sofia's parents had had enough of Sofia's nightly arrivals in their room, the musical beds, and the scrunched-up sleeping, and they were ready to help Sofia learn how to stay in her own bed all night. They worked through the five-step plan to address all of her needs around bedtime and prepared a plan for night wakings.

Sofia's mother stopped lying in Sofia's bed at bedtime and soon worked her way out of Sofia's room entirely. For the next three weeks, a parent had to bring Sofia back to her room each night after an awakening. They used a motion sensor on their master bedroom door so they would know exactly when Sofia came to their room each night. Soon Sofia was sleeping peacefully in her purple-canopied bed all night long, and her parents were sleeping peacefully (and fully stretched out) in their bed, too.

Luis, Who Kicked the TV Habit

Nine-year-old Luis fell asleep at 8 p.m. every night in his room with the TV on. His mother turned it off when she went to bed. His mother also slept with the TV on in her own room and, as she was a bit embarrassed to admit, had done so for years. Luis always woke up a few hours later, and, when he found his TV off, he either turned it back on in his own room or slipped into his mother's bed to watch TV in her room.

Both Luis and his mom had a sleep onset association with the TV and could fall asleep easily with it on, but they could not fall back to sleep once it was off. This sleep crutch was resulting in some sleep deprivation for Luis, and his mother also worried that he would not be able to sleep at a friend's home or at camp that upcoming summer without it.

His mother decided to help Luis learn to fall asleep without the TV. She also decided she should learn to kick the TV habit, too, so that Luis would not be tempted to come to her room at night to watch it there either!

She began the process by turning down the volume and the brightness on the TV both in his and her room, bit by bit, over a two-week period until she could turn the TV completely off in both places. She added a small nightlight to Luis's room and taught him to read himself to sleep each night. She enjoyed getting recommendations from his school librarians for books that nine-year-old boys were likely to enjoy, and she would read in a cozy chair nearby at the same time.

Once Luis could read himself to sleep easily, she removed the TV entirely from both of their rooms. Luis was soon sleeping through the night (and his mom learned to kick the habit and read herself to sleep each night, too!).

Tamar, Who Was a Great Sleeper
Until a Family Vacation

Eight-year-old Tamar was a great sleeper with a consistent and wonderful bedtime routine. She was a great sleeper, that is, until her family of five went on vacation and stayed in a relative's home for ten days. There were only two beds for the five of them, so Tamar, her little sister, and her mom slept in one bed, and Tamar's brother and dad slept in the other.

When the family returned home, Tamar cried at bedtime on the first night back and insisted that she and her sister should get to sleep in her mother's bed. Tamar, while on vacation, had quickly learned some new sleep onset associations, and she did not want to go back to her old sleep habits when she got home again. However, Tamar's mother had noticed that Tamar was a much more wakeful and restless sleeper when they were all together in one bed, and she knew that Tamar's sleep would be best if Tamar returned to her usual consistent routine. Tamar was soon back to being a great solo sleeper again once they began consistently using her 5B Bedtime Routine again each night.

Chloe, Who Would Fall Asleep Only for Her Mom

Chloe had never been a good sleeper. Although she was a third grader, she had been sleeping with her single mother every night since she was a baby. She was clingy and fearful during the day, as well, with a lot of trouble separating from her mother then, too.

Her mother, wanting to do everything she could to help Chloe feel less anxious whenever possible, did not initially want to help Chloe learn to become an independent sleeper. She felt that if she did not give Chloe everything she needed at bedtime and did not keep her close by when Chloe was anxious, she was not being a good mother. Chloe's mother had even been accepted to graduate school, but she had decided not to go because she didn't feel that she could leave Chloe with her aunt or grandmother to be put to bed in the evening.

Sleep issues often go hand-in-hand with anxiety and daytime separation issues. Some children who have these types of issues become much more confident and comfortable in their daytime settings once they become independent sleepers. Chloe's mother (without meaning to, of course) had been sending Chloe a message for a long time that Chloe was not capable of the skills that other third graders had mastered long ago.

Rather than helping Chloe, the support Chloe's mother had been providing was actually keeping Chloe from feeling self-reliant enough to do the things other girls her age were enjoying, such as sleepovers at a friend's or relative's home. This pattern was also getting in the way of Chloe's mother pursuing her own goals and obtaining the additional education that would have made her career more satisfying and their small family much more secure financially.

Chloe's mother decided she was ready to help Chloe become a better sleeper. First, Chloe's mother worked out a plan to very, very gradually taper herself out of Chloe's room at bedtime. First, she set up a spare bed in Chloe's room and started sleeping in this spare bed each night. As time went on, she moved this bed farther and farther away from Chloe until the bed was in the hallway. Then she eliminated the spare bed and sat in a chair in the hall as Chloe fell asleep. Over time, Chloe's mother was able to sleep in her own bedroom again.

At the same time, she began having Chloe's aunt and grandmother come over two or three nights each week to put Chloe to bed and, later still, Chloe began having sleepovers at their homes, too. Once Chloe had adjusted to these changes, Chloe's mom enrolled in graduate school and two years later, Chloe along with her aunt and grandmother had a very proud day watching Chloe's mother walk across the stage at her graduation ceremony.

Lola, Who Put Two Lawyers on Lockdown

Seven-year-old Lola was a very smart, spirited, and strong-willed girl whose parents were both attorneys. Over time and through many bedtime struggles, Lola had managed to convince her parents she needed both of them to be present and upstairs at bedtime. Lola wanted her mother to be with her in Lola's twin bed, and Lola wanted her father to be sitting on the bed in the master bedroom where Lola could see him if she sat up and looked down the hall. Neither parent was allowed to be downstairs until Lola was fast asleep! Moreover, neither of Lola's parents ever left their home in the evening for any reason, and they were missing out on many social engagements, gym workouts, and community meetings. This was affecting their careers and friendships as well as their health and their marital relationship.

Lola's parents were frustrated with the "Lola Lockdown" and were ready to design a new bedtime routine for her. As part of the new plan, they decided that one parent each night would be completely out of the house or, at a minimum, downstairs in the living room or kitchen. The parent on duty for that night finished up the bedtime routine and then moved to a chair in Lola's room to read. This parent reminded Lola that she could read or play quietly in her bed until she was drowsy enough to go to sleep and that he or she would stay nearby until she did.

At first, Lola often did some long and loud protesting the moment the parent on duty moved to the chair and the other parent left. Each time this happened, Lola's mom or dad moved to the doorway and repeated a variation of the broken record statement described in Chapter 7 that is used if a child becomes disruptive at bedtime. The broken record statement that Lola's parents used was, "I am your parent, and this is the new bedtime plan. I will only sit in your room if you are quiet and in bed."

Lola's parents alternated who put her to bed each night. They continued step by step with a gradual tapering of their presence in her room, and after some initial setbacks and some bumps in the road (during which they made sure to stay very consistent with the rules) they were eventually freed from the "Lola Lockdown."

Theodora, Who Had the Sleep Schedule of a Teenager

Four-year-old Theodora fell asleep very late at night (usually between 11 p.m. and midnight). She woke up for the day around 11 a.m. She went to preschool at noon so her mother and father did not initially have a problem with this sleep schedule. They also liked this schedule because they both worked late, and her grandmother stayed at their house and played with Theodora until both of her parents got home from work. They liked to spend time with Theodora before they all went to bed around midnight.

However, Theodora's parents were beginning to worry about her sleep schedule because Theodora was going to be attending kindergarten in the fall. They decided to begin shifting her sleep schedule so she could get up at 8 a.m. by the time school started. The first week, they started by getting her up each day a half hour earlier than usual, at 10:30 a.m. They made sure she had some sunlight exposure after she woke up by taking her across the street to the playground right after giving her breakfast and getting her dressed. Sunlight exposure, activity, and a meal help to "set" the rise time of a child's internal clock. Every week or two, they moved her rise time back by a half hour or so until they reached the desired rise time of 8 a.m. Lola was rested and ready to go each morning by the time school started that year.

Levi, Who Wanted to Go to Summer Camp

Nine-year-old Levi really, really wanted to go to camp with his friends during the upcoming summer. January, February, and March came and went, and his family still had not sent in the deposit and paperwork. Both Levi and his parents were worried he would not be able to sleep well at camp because he had a hard time falling asleep each night, even in his own home. He always needed one of his parents to sit in a beanbag chair in his room at night until he was deeply asleep. His room was dim, and it was hard to see the beanbag chair, so he often sat up and checked to make sure either his mother or his father was still nearby. Each night, it took Levi more than two hours to fall asleep.

Levi's parents decided to help him learn to read himself to sleep every night. They continued to sit in a beanbag chair in his room, and they gave Levi the kind of reading light that had a small headlamp on an adjustable headband. When his bedtime routine was over, he lay in bed reading with his reading light until he fell asleep each night. His parents began to work their way out of his room gradually, too. It didn't take long until Levi was telling his parents they could leave his room right after the bedtime routine was over. Levi felt so confident about being able to read himself to sleep each night that his parents were soon able to sign him up for summer camp!

Phoebe, Who Was a Nighttime Screamer

Five-year-old Phoebe had difficulty falling asleep at night and difficulty staying asleep. Phoebe's mom read three books with Phoebe and then left her room each night. However, Phoebe made many callbacks and curtain calls after her mom left, and it took her a long time to transition into sleep.

Once Phoebe was asleep, she slept for several hours, but once she awakened, she ran screaming down the hall to her mother's side of the bed. She refused to go back to her room at all at that time of the night and would not fall back to sleep unless she was lying on top of her mother in the master bed where she stayed the rest of the night.

Many parents think if they are out of their child's room when the child actually falls asleep, their child will not have any sleep issues during the night. However, parents often do not realize that being able to make many callbacks and curtain calls is, actually, also a kind of sleep crutch. These parent-child interactions happen over and over around bedtime until the child is finally drowsy enough to fall asleep. But when this child awakens, he or she needs more of these interactions again even though he or she fell asleep alone in his or her room at bedtime. This type of sleep difficulty can be improved by using Bedtime Tickets and by choosing ahead of time how night wakings will be handled.

Phoebe's mother began giving Phoebe two Bedtime Tickets each night and then reminded her to read or play until she was drowsy enough to fall asleep. If Phoebe screamed in the night and came to her mother's room, her mother walked her back each time whether or not Phoebe protested and sat in a chair in Phoebe's doorway until she was asleep again.

Phoebe's nocturnal screaming soon resolved, and she fell asleep much more quickly at bedtime, too.

Aidan, Who Needed a Sleep Study

Seven-year-old Aidan snored and made gasping sounds at night that worried his parents. Aidan also had some attention and behavioral issues in the daytime at school, and his teachers recommended he have an evaluation for ADHD. However, Aidan's pediatrician wisely recommended a sleep study first to rule out any type of medical sleep disorder, such as sleep apnea, that might result in the type of poor sleep that would also cause daytime issues with attention and behavior.

Aidan's parents worked hard to prepare him for the sleep study, especially because he had some sensory processing issues. They did four things to prepare him:

- They watched an online instructional video about pediatric sleep studies several times to help Aidan understand what would happen on the night of the study.

- They visited the sleep center during the daytime for a tour and to see the room Aidan would sleep in. There was a cabinet with new toys in the sleep center, and they showed Aidan that he would be going home with a new toy once the sleep study was finished.

- They talked with the sleep center psychologist about how to "desensitize" Aidan at home before arriving on the study night (see Appendix A).

- They put together a bag with items that would make the sleep study night easier for Aidan (see Appendix A).

Aidan practiced doing a sleep study setup on his mother and on his favorite stuffed animal, and then his father did a practice setup on Aidan. This helped Aidan to have an easy experience on the night of the study and a successful outcome.

The sleep study did show that Aidan had sleep apnea, and after talking to an ENT (ear, nose, and throat) physician who had been recommended by Aidan's pediatrician, Aidan had his tonsils and adenoids removed. He began sleeping very deeply again, and his attention and behavior issues completely resolved.

APPENDIX A

How to Prepare Your Child
for a Sleep Study

What Is a Sleep Study?
And Why Do Some Children Need One?

A sleep study is an overnight test that measures several things that happen during a child's sleep. A sleep study is often used to rule out some type of medical sleep disorder such as sleep apnea.

What Is Involved in a Sleep Study?

A sleep study requires that a technician do a "setup" on your child at the beginning of the night. The setup takes about one hour, and your child can watch a video or read a book during this time. None of the sensations that occur during the setup cause any pain, but they can be hard for some children to adjust to. The setup might involve the following:

- electrodes (small metal disks) are applied with a washable paste to the scalp (to determine what kind of sleep your child is getting) and to the face on either side of the eyes (to find out how much dream sleep your child achieves)

- a stretchy "hat" made out of gauze is wrapped around the head (to hold the electrodes on your child's scalp in place)

- an electrode is placed on the chest over the heart (to monitor your child's heart rate and rhythm) and sometimes on the legs (to track the number of limb movements your child makes at night and determine whether these wake him or her)

- a bandage-style sensor is wrapped around a toe or finger (to monitor your child's oxygen level)

- a stretchy belt is wrapped around the chest and another one is wrapped around the abdomen (to monitor your child's breathing effort)

- soft plastic prongs are placed in the nostrils (this is called a nasal cannula), and a flow sensor is taped under the nose (to monitor the flow of air coming in and out of your child's nose)

- a small microphone is taped to the neck (to listen for snoring)

How Can I Prepare
My Child for a Sleep Study?

If you are interested in spending some time at home before the sleep study to help your child get used to these sensations (this is called doing a "desensitization"), your child may have a much easier time the night of the study and be able to achieve more sleep. Most sleep centers will give you a take-home kit with some of the items that will be used for the sleep study, and you can assemble the rest from a drugstore. You will need the following items:

- soft surgical tape (the kind that peels off easily and feels like cloth)

- a roll of 2-inch-wide gauze

- a regular adhesive bandage

- a roll of cotton elastic bandages

- a few stick-on electrodes and a nasal cannula. The sleep center where your child will have the study is often willing to give you these last two items if you stop in and request them.

Once you have collected these items, practice doing a sleep study setup on yourself while your child watches, as follows:

- Put some small pieces of tape on various places on the top of your head to mimic the attachment of the electrodes.

- Wrap some gauze around your head to keep the pieces of tape in place. Try calling it a "ninja hat" or some other type of hat that would appeal to your child.

- Wrap an adhesive bandage around your finger or toe to mimic the oxygen sensor.

- Wrap wide elastic bandages around your chest and stomach to mimic the two respiratory-effort belts.

- Place the soft nasal cannula prongs into your nose and put a tiny piece of tape below your nose to hold it in place. Wrap the extra tubing behind your ears and cut off any extra plastic tubing.

- Stick an electrode pad onto your chest by your heart and onto your legs.

During all of this, model calmness and comfort. Your child can then re-use these items to do a sleep study setup on you or on his or her favorite stuffed animal. Lastly, you can do a practice sleep study setup on your child at home, adding each item one at a time (and perhaps working on this over several days). Always combine this practice with an activity your child enjoys (for example, having a snack or listening to your child's favorite music).

While you are working on this, try to repeat key phrases such as: "Only an adult puts these items on, and only an adult takes these items off" and "These items might tickle but they don't hurt."

The nasal cannula is often the most difficult item to adjust to and one that a child might try to pull off. When you put the nasal cannula on your child, be aware that it is especially important to help your child practice wearing the nasal cannula only while something positive is happening. For example, you might take some cookies out of the oven and put the nasal cannula on your child before he or she is given a warm cookie. Or perhaps if your child wants to watch a new video, you might let your child watch it only while wearing the nasal cannula for a period of time.

If your child does try to take the cannula off once you have put it on him or her, you can very briefly remove the positive thing your child likes (for example, by pausing the video for a moment or by waiting to give your child a second cookie) until your child allows you to replace the nasal cannula again.

Since these items will be presented gradually while being associated only with positive things, your child will very likely feel much calmer and more comfortable when he or she sees these items again in the sleep center during the sleep study setup.

What to Bring
on the Night of the Sleep Study

Most sleep centers will ask you to bring the following items:

- insurance card and parent's photo identification

- two-piece sleepwear that is loose and comfortable. Cotton is preferred but not necessary.

- socks or slippers

- favorite pillow, blanket, or stuffed toy

- medications

- snacks for nighttime and for the next morning

What to Do on the
Day of the Sleep Study

There are some things a child can do to help ensure that the study night is more likely to go well:

- follow a normal sleep routine during the day or two prior to the study

- avoid taking a long nap on the day of the study

- avoid caffeine (such as chocolate or soda) for forty-eight hours prior to the study

- eat dinner before arriving

- arrive bathed and with clean hair (no gels, hairspray, or other oily substances)

Frequently Asked Questions About the Five-Step Plan

● **What should my child use for a Bedtime Buddy if he never chose a security object?**

If your child never developed an attachment to a security object such as a stuffed bear, blanket, or lovey, this may be because your child has almost always had *you* nearby as a security object to help with the transition into sleep! If you want to try to help your child bond to a security object, you can encourage your child to choose one of his stuffed animals (or even take your child shopping for a special new one), and then you can begin including this animal every night in the bedtime routine. If your child just doesn't want a Bedtime Buddy, though, this is not essential.

Lukas chose a stuffed tiger cub as his Bedtime Buddy. Tiger began coming along for the ride during every part of the bedtime routine. For example, Tiger sat at the kitchen table while Lukas had his bedtime snack, he sat on the edge of the bathtub at bedtime, and he read books with Lukas and his parents until reading time was over. Then, Lukas played with Tiger and other quiet toys from his Bedtime Basket in bed until he was drowsy enough to fall asleep on his own. When Lukas woke up at night, Tiger was still nearby to cuddle.

What if I've tried this type of approach before and my child never learned how to self-comfort?

If you have tried this approach before without success, think back carefully to what you did. Did you let your child cry and then eventually give up and do what you had always done to help him or her get to sleep (instead of giving your child the space to learn how to fall asleep when you were nearby but quiet)?

Did you give up after one or two difficult nights, perhaps just when your child was on the verge of making some progress? Did you give up because you were worried that your child might lose too much sleep? Remember that your child will take longer at first to fall asleep when you are sleep coaching him, but he will soon be getting much *more* sleep. And if your child needed sleep coaching in the first place, your child was probably already losing some sleep.

If you wanted to learn to sleep without a pillow, you would need to try to fall asleep each and every night without it. This would take some time, of course, but if someone brought you a pillow after you had spent some time trying to learn this new skill, you would never learn how to do it, and you would be right back to square one.

● **What if my child makes a curtain call after the Bedtime Tickets are gone or have expired?**

Remember that this behavior is part of your child's attempt to avoid learning the skill of falling asleep independently. If your child makes a curtain call after the Bedtime Tickets are gone or have expired, calmly and quickly guide your child back to bed each time with minimal interaction, touching, or eye contact. Repeat the broken record phrase **"Your Bedtime Tickets are gone. Please read or play until you are sleepy. It's bedtime."** Then, quickly leave again.

If your child has a hard time remembering to stay in his or her room, you can try hanging a homemade paper stop sign in the doorway as a reminder. Some children even need a gate (or perhaps the type of door latch that allows the door to be opened only a few inches) to remind them.

● **Should I ever lock my child in his or her room?**

Never! This is very frightening for a child and completely unnecessary.

● **What if my child throws a tantrum when the bedtime routine is over?**

Your child may test you a great deal the first few nights to make sure that you really plan to stick with the new routine. Your child may throw a tantrum (or more than one!). This is completely normal and is sometimes called an "extinction burst." This means that when you are expecting a new behavior from your child and getting rid of an old one, he or she may increase negative behaviors temporarily in an attempt to get you to change your mind.

All children have behaviors they use to get you to change your mind about something. Your child might whine or cry very loudly. He or she might throw things. Your child might try to do something that could be dangerous. He or she might call you a "mean mom." Your child might sweetly ask you to lie down with him or her for "just one minute" or tell you in a shaky voice that he or she just glimpsed a scary monster. These behaviors will all soon decrease if you are calm, firm, and consistent. These behaviors are often more frequent on the second night of a new routine than on the first, by the way. Even once things are going well, most children will test you again a few nights later.

● **Should I try the Bedtime Delay Technique?**

Perhaps. When you start this process, you may want to *temporarily* move your child's bedtime to the time that your child is actually falling asleep now (even if this is as late as 10 p.m., for example). This is called the bedtime delay technique. Starting the routine later often helps things to move along quickly because your child may be so tired that he or she may be able to fall asleep quickly, even with the new routine. You are essentially trying to increase the chance of quick success with the new routine. Once your child is falling asleep quickly, move the bedtime back by fifteen minutes every few days or so until you arrive back at a more appropriate bedtime. The bedtime delay is not a good choice for every child, however. Some children become even more active the later it gets at night.

Should my spouse (or partner) and I take turns doing the routine?

Yes. Be sure that both you and your spouse or partner, if possible, take turns doing the bedtime routine. It's important to teach your child to accept either caregiver at bedtime so one of you can leave home in the evening if you need or want to, and so both of you learn how to follow the routine consistently. Don't worry if the routine is different when your child is away from home occasionally (for example, at a relative's or step-parent's home). Children can learn that there are one set of rules at home and another when they are away. The most important thing is to be consistent in the place where the child spends the most time.

If your child asks for your spouse when it is your night, be very matter-of-fact and say something like, "It's Dad's night tonight, and tomorrow it will be Mom's night." If he or she continues to ask, you could try saying something like, "It's Dad's night or no one's . . ." Don't give in!

● **How do I know if my child really needs me when the routine is over and I've left the room?**

Children do, of course, sometimes have very legitimate needs after the bedtime routine ends. They might think that something is wrong with a sibling or pet, or they might worry that something is wrong in the house (for example, they might hear an unusual sound or smell something strange). These are things that you should, of course, teach them to report to you, even if the routine is over and the Bedtime Tickets have been used or have expired. If the need doesn't seem legitimate once you have checked it out, just quickly return to the plan.

● **What if my child becomes ill during the night?**

Teach your child to come and tell you right away if he or she feels ill, feverish, or nauseous during the night. Your child should know that he or she can call out or come to you in these situations and be reminded that he or she doesn't need a Bedtime Ticket for this.

● **What if my child has to go to the bathroom during the night? What if my child is potty training and still needs my help after the bedtime routine is over?**

If your child is already potty trained, he or she should be allowed to go to the bathroom alone without an interaction with you at bedtime and reminded that a Bedtime Ticket isn't necessary for this. It may help to provide a small reward the first few times your child does this. If your child is very young and you think your child might need an interim step, try putting a portable potty in your child's room at night near a nightlight so that he or she does not have to leave the room. This is also useful if your child makes a game of calling you back frequently at bedtime to take him or her to the bathroom. Most children become a lot less interested in going to the bathroom if they don't get an escorted trip from mom and dad. If your child is still potty training and still needs your help, simply go to your child and quietly help him or her and then leave again.

- **Do I have to be consistent every night?**
Can we take a break on the weekends?

Consistency makes this process much easier for your child. The most common problem for families who seek help with bedtime problems is a lack of consistency. Their children do not know what to expect and cannot settle down easily at night because of this. Being consistent and doing each step in the 5B Bedtime Routine in the same order every night helps your child become a great sleeper much more rapidly.

Giving in to protests after a period of time makes the process even harder on your child. If you are firm for the first thirty minutes and then give in to your child, you are teaching your child to cry and act out for a long period until you cave in. If you are firm one night and then give in on another night, this will be confusing and frustrating for your child. When you decide to teach your child to fall asleep independently, you must be willing to follow through consistently. Giving in *some of the time* is the quickest way to make this process take longer.

What if my child cries when the bedtime routine is over?

Some parents have no difficulty setting limits if a child cries or protests about something during the daytime, but these same parents sometimes have much more trouble doing so at bedtime. For example, most parents would never allow their child to play with matches, run in a parking lot, have lots of sugary snacks before dinner, or decide whether or not to have a bath. If their child complained or cried about these daytime rules, they would just ignore these protests. If you agree that daytime rules are important, then you can leave behind any guilt about a gentle, age-appropriate bedtime routine with nighttime rules!

Long spells of crying are *not* a necessary part of teaching your child to become an independent sleeper. This book details a very gentle and gradual way of helping your child accomplish this skill. However, remember that just a few minutes of protest crying or fussing around bedtime will not do any permanent harm to your child. You already know this because, as we talked about above, you already ignore some protest crying when you set limits in the daytime. For example, if your child cried because you served juice instead of soda, or if you made her wear a bike helmet, you would not let that short period of protest crying change your mind about your decision.

You are accomplishing something very useful and important when you teach your child how to fall asleep independently, so try not to let a little protest crying deter you. Try to think of this as giving your child the space he or she needs to learn this new skill.

Your child will show great improvement in only two or three nights if you are consistent. Clear limits are actually very comforting for your child. Remember that you can't *make* your child go to sleep, but you can remind your child of the task at hand. Each time you say the broken record phrase you learned in Chapter 7 (**"Your Bedtime Tickets are gone. Read or play until you are sleepy. It's bedtime."**), you remind your child of the task at hand: playing quietly in bed until he or she is ready to fall asleep.

Some parents like to have phrases that they can keep in mind when the going gets tough. If you think you would benefit from this, try choosing one or two of these phrases:

• "By working my way out of my child's room, I'm sending the message that my child is safe without me. Sleeping alone is not dangerous or traumatic but instead often leads to the best and most restful sleep."

- "If my child cries while I'm sitting quietly nearby, I'm not ignoring crying. I'm staying close by while allowing my child the space she needs to learn how to fall asleep independently."

- "Setting limits sends an important message to my child: sometimes my child has to do things he doesn't want to do, and sometimes my child doesn't get his way. I don't want to teach my child that crying or throwing a tantrum will work to get what he wants."

- "Sitting supportively and silently nearby is often the wisest and most effective response to protesting, bargaining, yelling, and crying."

- "My child is old enough to sleep in his own bed without me now. I will help him, and he will be fine. I'll be nearby, even when I'm not in his room. He has his place to sleep, and I have mine."

- "My child will do better in so many ways if I teach her to be a great sleeper. She will be able to sleep away from home at a friend's or relative's home or at summer camp. I am a loving parent to teach my child this skill."

● **Will this new bedtime routine cause psychological trauma or other problems for my child?**

Many parents have some concerns about the process of teaching their child how to fall asleep quickly and independently. If this is true for you, the information below may help. First, remember that you should feel free to move as slowly as you like while you are tapering your presence (as reviewed in Chapter 6).

If you are worried your child will feel abandoned or alone when you leave the bedroom or if you fear you might be ignoring your child's legitimate needs at bedtime, remember that a well-thought out, consistent bedtime routine with one or two Bedtime Tickets for additional requests makes this very unlikely. The routine and tickets are designed to make sure all of a child's most important needs are met.

Your child will learn that you will always provide for these needs but that you are not willing to allow interactions with you to go on indefinitely after the bedtime routine ends because this leads to lost sleep. Your child will also learn that you are not going to offer unnecessary support after addressing his or her needs.

You can have lots of special time during the day with your child, but at the end of the day, it's time for a comforting, consistent routine that allows your child to fall asleep quickly. As long as you provide plenty of love and attention during the day and during each of the steps in your bedtime routine, your child will soon be thriving and sleeping better and you will, too!

If you are worried that setting limits at bedtime will cause some sort of psychological damage to your child, consider how you feel about setting daytime limits. You probably have no guilt about having firm and non-negotiable limits in the daytime (for example, no playing with matches, no yelling in a restaurant, and no avoiding a bath when needed). So, if you don't spend much time during the day worrying whether limit setting will cause long-term damage to your child, remember that you should not worry about gentle, consistent, predictable nighttime limit setting either.

If you are worried your child will not like the new bedtime routine, remember that many children (and most people, for that matter) tend not to like change, so your child indeed may not like some of these changes at first. However, your child's current routine is probably leading to sleep deprivation for your child and for you and your family as well. This pattern may also be causing some daytime behavioral problems.

Your child does not always understand what is best for him or her in the long run. There is a difference between responding to a legitimate need at bedtime and letting things get out of control. Loving your child doesn't mean letting him or her have all the power. You can set limits for your child to be sure everyone in your home gets the sleep they need and still be a very nurturing and loving parent. These two goals are definitely not mutually exclusive!

If you are worried that setting limits at bedtime will make your child feel *less close* to you, remember your child will actually feel *more safe and secure* around you when he or she can predict what you will do at bedtime. Parents often get angry around bedtime when the routine isn't working well, and this can be much more upsetting for your child. The predictability of this bedtime routine is actually likely to be very comforting for your child over the long run and will usually help your child feel much more trusting toward you. Your child no longer has to worry about whether the preferred parent will be home each night at bedtime, or whether that parent will be calm and loving or irritable and short-tempered at bedtime.

If you are worried that the new bedtime routine will make your child anxious, remember that anxiety around bedtime most often means a child does not yet know how to fall asleep without parental assistance. It also often indicates the current routine does not have consistent limits, and this may increase a child's anxiety.

If you are the type of parent who likes to review the research about the effects of sleep training, you may be interested in reviewing a study that followed up on children five years after they had been sleep trained. This study found there were no negative impacts on these children's mental health or on the relationship between these children and their parents.*

- **What if I am concerned that my child might yell or cry during this process and wake or upset my other children?**

You will want to share with your other children the reasons why you are helping this child learn to be a great sleeper. You may also need to temporarily let a sibling sleep elsewhere if this child is protesting a lot at the beginning of this process.

---

*A. M. Price, M. Wake, O. C. Ukoumunne, and H. Hiscock, "Five-year follow-up of harms and benefits of behavioral infant sleep intervention: randomized trial," *Pediatrics* 130, no. 4 (2012): 643–651.

● **What if I am concerned that my child might yell or cry during this process and upset my live-in relatives? Or upset the neighbors that live in the apartment next to mine?**

Be sure to read the story about Grace in the Epilogue. You may want to share your plans with these people. Express your confidence that you are doing something very important for your child (and review with them some of the reasons covered in Chapter 3). You could even show them a copy of this book.

● **Should my child have his or her own bed? Or can my child share a bed with a sibling?**

It's best to have your child sleep in his or her own bed each night, but it is fine for siblings to share a room. Even the simplest and smallest bed is best for learning to fall asleep independently and being able to handle sleepovers or summer camp without any issues. Studies show that adults and children who sleep alone have fewer awakenings and change positions less often than those who sleep with someone. Sleeping alone is not something to be avoided and often results in better sleep.

- **What if I have more than one child with sleep problems?**

You may have more than one child who needs your sleep-coaching skills. If so, you could choose one child to start with and, once that child is sleeping well, move on to another child. However, if you have good support at bedtime and think it would be easier to start using the five-step plan in this book for all of your preschool and school-age children at the same time, you should feel free to do so. Just be sure to think about how you will use the five-step plan for each child (preparing his or her bedroom, choosing his or her Bedtime Buddy, filling a Bedtime Basket with items he or she could use, making a 5B Bedtime Routine chart that fits his or her age and preferences, and so on).

- **What if my child asks to drink milk or eat during the night or sneaks into the kitchen to get food once I fall asleep?**

Be sure to read the story about Oliver, the midnight snacker, in the Epilogue. Try to avoid allowing your child to eat (or drink anything except water) after the bedtime routine concludes or during the night. If you do, your child's "stomach alarm clock" may begin waking your child up at the same time every night to eat. A child's nutritional needs should be met with good meals throughout the day and a substantial, satisfying, and healthy bedtime snack. If, despite your best efforts, your child waits until you are asleep and then slips into the kitchen to eat, you may need to talk to your child's pediatrician or a nutritionist.

● **Should my child have a consistent rise time, even if he or she did not get much sleep the night before due to the new routine?**

Yes. Think about what time you want your child to get up each day. Then choose a bedtime that would allow for the age-appropriate number of hours for sleep (see Chapter 1). A 6 a.m. rise time would mean an 8–9 p.m. bedtime, for example, depending on the age of the child. A consistent rise time also helps your child become sleepy at the appropriate time the next night. Allowing your child to sleep in often may keep your child from having a strong sleep drive at the appropriate bedtime.

How can I help my child wake up more easily in the morning and feel alert at school?

If you want to help your child wake up more easily in the morning, keep your child's rise time consistent seven days a week. The body makes up for sleep lost on one night by increasing the percentage of deep and dream sleep the very next night, so catching up the next night or on the weekend isn't usually necessary. If your child does sleep in late each weekend to catch up on sleep, for example, he or she often won't be sleepy again at the desired bedtime on Sunday night because he or she won't have been awake long enough.

To help your child feel as alert as possible at school, try helping your child get some sunlight exposure before going into the school building, perhaps by getting to the bus stop a little early or by having breakfast outdoors on your porch or deck if the weather allows. If you help your child obtain exposure to sunlight at about the same time each morning, this helps to set your child's internal clock for the appropriate rise time. Sunlight is also a free, healthy, and powerful stimulant for the brain and helps your child to fully wake up.

Having breakfast each morning will also help your child be more alert and awake at school. Try to include some protein in whatever your child chooses for breakfast. If your child doesn't like to eat breakfast, a smoothie with some protein powder or a handful of nuts might be a good choice.

The Printable 5B Bedtime Chart and Bedtime Tickets

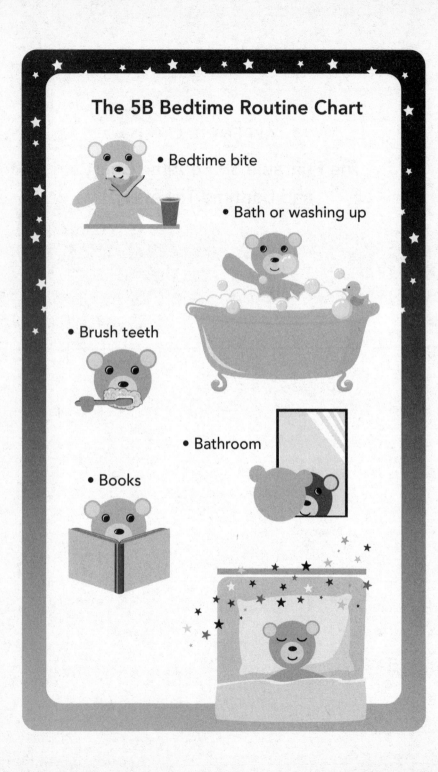

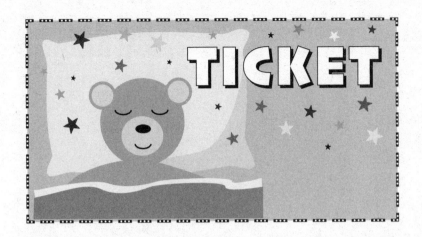

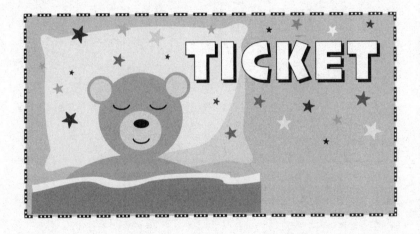

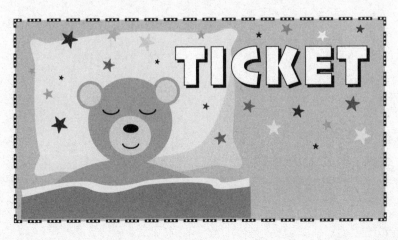

Acknowledgments

I want to first express my gratitude to my treasured PCCSM and Psychiatry colleagues at the Yale School of Medicine and at the Yale Centers for Sleep Medicine (especially Meir Kryger, MD, who generously offered his counsel during the writing of this book) and at Connecticut Children's Medical Center (especially Jay Kenkare, MD, who has been a steady source of support and wisdom). I am fortunate to call these people my friends as well as my colleagues.

I also want to thank Linda Konner, my literary agent, for her wise guidance; Dan Ambrosio, my editor, whose insight and vision structured and shaped this book; and all the other kind and knowledgeable people at Hachette Book Group including Anna Hall, Miriam Riad, Michael Barrs, and Amanda Kain. Many thanks also to Lori Hobkirk of the Book Factory who guided me so surely through the production process.

I would be much less savvy about social media without the upbeat and skilled folks at Zilker Media (Rusty Shelton, Paige Velasquez, Nichole Williamson, and Alexis Crowell).

I am so grateful to the diverse, talented, and supportive faculty at Harvard Medical School's annual "Writing, Publishing, and Social Media for Healthcare Professionals" course where this book became a reality (especially the phenomenal course director, Julie Silver, MD, and the very talented book coach, Lisa Tener) and to the inspiring and creative friends I reconnect with there each year.

I am fortunate to have many brilliant and inspirational people in my circle of family and friends. Among them are the Young Quilters, the O'Mamas, the Zeteos, my SCC and TUCW friends, my book club gals, and my friends in Lake Hills, Fairfield, and beyond. Suzanne, Robin, Whitney, Mary, Lynda, Susan gave me such great support and guidance. I'd like to especially thank Wendy for so kindly reviewing many versions of this book and for always being so generous with her sage advice. I also want to express my deep gratitude to my parents and to my wonderful Schneeberg, Fulda, Bell, and Browne families. Each of you enrich my life in innumerable ways.

Above all, my everlasting thanks to my husband, Gordon, and to our beautiful children, William, Evelynne, and Marie. You fill my life with joy, support, and love.

Index

About the Author

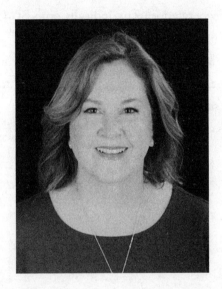

Once people at a social gathering find out that Dr. Lynelle Schneeberg treats childhood sleep problems for a living, groups of exhausted parents eager for help gather around her.

Dr. Schneeberg, also known as the Bedtime Doctor, is a behavioral sleep psychologist who has helped thousands of families solve their children's sleep problems. She is an assistant professor at the Yale School of Medicine and the director of the Behavioral Sleep Program at Connecticut Children's Medical Center. She is also a Fellow of the

American Academy of Sleep Medicine. Because her evidence-based plan has worked so well, parents and colleagues suggested she write a book in order to share her secrets with a wider audience.

Dr. Schneeberg appears periodically on NBC Connecticut and on Fox 61 in its "Ask the Bedtime Doctor" segments to discuss a variety of childhood sleep issues. She is frequently invited to speak to healthcare professionals and to the public on a variety of childhood sleep topics.